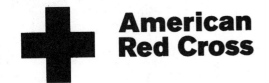

American Red Cross

Emergency Response Workbook

StayWell

StayWell
263 Summer Street
Boston, MA 02210

International Standard Book Number 1–8151–1273–4

00 01 02 03 / 9   8   7   6   5

Contents

Introduction

This workbook is designed to accompany the American Red Cross—Emergency Response textbook. Specific workbook activities were created to help you review the most important material in the text, to help you practice making appropriate decisions about emergency care, and to help you prepare for the skills and written evaluation. The material in each unit of this workbook reinforces key concepts and skills taught in the textbook. This affords you the opportunity to build on learned material and apply your knowledge to emergency situations. Most of the workbook activities allow you to work at your own pace and evaluate your progress at various stages.

To maximize the benefit of using the Emergency Response Workbook, you are encouraged to first read the textbook, then answer the questions in the corresponding unit of this workbook. You may need to reference your textbook for questions you are unable to answer. After completing the activities in each unit, check you answers against those at the end of this workbook. For help with those questions that you answered incorrectly or with difficulty, return to the corresponding chapter in the textbook, and review the relevant material. If you still do not understand why an answer is correct or have additional questions about the material you are studying, ask your instructor for help.

In each unit of the workbook you will find the following sections:

◆ Summary

This section summarizes the key concepts and ideas presented in the corresponding chapter of the textbook.

◆ Outline

The outline lists the major headings and subheadings of the textbook chapter. Use the outline as a reference when looking for a specific topic in a chapter.

◆ Learning Activities

This section is the heart of the workbook. It contains a variety of activities that test and reinforce your understanding and retention of the material in the textbook. The activities in this section consist of—
◆ Matching exercises.
◆ True/False questions.
◆ Short answer questions.
◆ Labeling exercises.

◆ Case Studies

In the Case Studies, found in most units, descriptions are given of specific emergency scenarios followed by questions that ask how you, as a first responder, would react to these situations and what care you would provide. These questions challenge you to apply the information you have learned to problems and situations you are likely to encounter, and help you develop logical solutions.

◆ Self-Assessment

Each workbook unit contains ten multiple choice questions on the material in the corresponding chapter of the textbook. These exercises give you practical experience in answering multiple choice questions and help prepare you for the final written examination given at the end of this course.

◆ Skill Sheets

Some units also contain skill sheets. These skill sheets identify the skills you should be able to demonstrate to your instructor at the end of the chapter in the textbook that describes them. The skill sheets contain illustrations and simple step-by-step directions on how to perform each skill. Have the appropriate sheets with you when you practice a particular skill.

Completing these workbook exercises as you progress through the textbook will help enhance your comprehension of the material in this course.

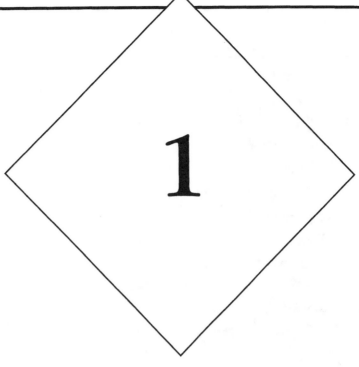

The First Responder

◆ SUMMARY

The survival and recovery of a severely ill or injured person depends on all parts of the emergency medical services (EMS) system working together efficiently. Citizen response, rapid activation of EMS, first responder care, advanced out-of-hospital emergency care, hospital care, and extended care (rehabilitation) are the links in this chain of survival. You, as a first responder, are often the first trained person to arrive on the emergency scene and take over care of the victim from any citizen responders present.

After arriving on the scene, the first responder checks the scene for safety and then reaches the victim, gives care for any life-threatening conditions, and summons more advanced medical personnel if needed. The first responder should give arriving medical personnel any assistance they need.

Regardless of your profession, when you are called upon to help a victim of injury or sudden illness, you assume the role of an emergency care provider. When an emergency occurs, the people in your care, as well as assisting bystanders, will expect you to know what to do. Be prepared to think and act accordingly. What to do, however, often involves more than giving emergency care. Chapter 19 provides an overview of the first responder's role in assessing and managing emergency scenes. In addition to caring for victims, first responders have a responsibility to maintain their health and stay up-to-date in their knowledge and training.

As emergency care providers, many first responders work under the supervision of a medical director. By planning in advance and following protocols and standing orders, out-of-hospital providers are able to perform certain skills and procedures through direct or indirect medical control.

◆ OUTLINE

◆ LEARNING ACTIVITIES

Matching

Match each term with its definition. Write its letter on the line in front of the definition.

Terms

a. Citizen responder

b. Emergency medical services (EMS) system

c. Emergency medical technician

d. First responder

e. Direct medical control

f. Indirect medical control

g. Medical director

h. Medical oversight

i. Protocols

j. Standing orders

Definitions

1. __B__ A person who has successfully completed a state-approved emergency care training program; paramedics are included in this group

2. __B__ A type of medical oversight in which the physician speaks directly with emergency care providers at the scene of an emergency

3. _____ A layperson who recognizes an emergency and decides to help

4. _____ The monitoring of care given by out-of-hospital providers to ill or injured victims, usually done by the medical director

5. _____ Standardized procedures to be followed when providing care to victims of illness or injury

6. _____ A network of community resources and medical personnel that provides emergency care to victims of injury or sudden illness

7. _____ A person, such as a police officer or fire fighter, trained in emergency care; the link between citizen responder care and advanced out-of-hospital care

8. _____ A type of medical oversight that includes education, protocol review, and quality improvement of emergency care providers

9. _____ Protocols issued by the medical director that allow specific skills to be performed or specific medications administered in certain situations

10. _____ A physician who assumes the responsibility for care of ill or injured victims in the out-of-hospital setting

True/False

Circle T if the statement is true; circle F if it is false.

1. (T) F   The first responder's role in the EMS system is identical to the role of the citizen responder.

2. T F   The goal of National Highway Traffic Safety Administration (NHTSA) of the U.S. Department of Transportation (DOT) is to reduce death and disabilities caused by motor vehicle crashes.

3. T F   The EMS system consists of community resources organized to care for victims of sudden illness or injury.

4. T F   Doing well in a first responder training program minimizes the need for continuing education, professional reading, and refresher training.

5. T F   Bringing rapid medical care to the victim rather than bringing the victim to medical care is a basic principle of the EMS system.

6. T F   The emergency medical technician is the next link in the chain of survival after the first responder.

7. T F   Keeping skills and knowledge up to date is an important characteristic of the first responder.

8. T F   The actions of the citizen responder represent the first crucial link in the EMS system.

9. T F   Each state has very specific laws and rules that govern the practice of EMS in the out-of-hospital setting.

Short Answer

Read each statement or question and write the correct answer or answers in the space provided.

1. The EMS system "chain of survival" links a series of events that improves outcomes for ill or injured victims. Write in the events that make up the links.

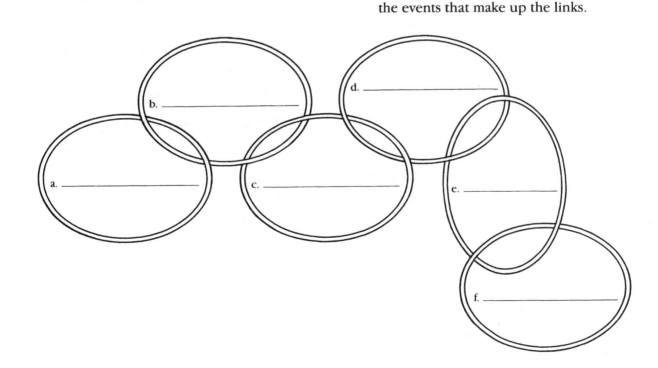

2. Effective first responders have certain characteristics that help them in their work. List at least three of these characteristics.

3. In 1973, the United States Congress enacted the Emergency Medical Services Act. What was the effect of this law?

4. NHTSA has created 10 components of an effective EMS system. List 6 of the 10 components.

5. How are direct medical control and indirect medical control the same, and how do they differ?

◆ SELF-ASSESSMENT

Circle the letter of the best answer.

1. Effective first responders have certain characteristics that help them in their work. Which of the following is one of those characteristics?

    a. Staying fit with daily exercise and a healthy diet

    b. Responding quickly and safely to the emergency scene

    c. Providing necessary emergency care

    d. Controlling all responders at the emergency scene

2. Indirect medical control includes all of the following types of medical oversight **except—**

    a. Off-line.

    b. Retrospective.

    c. On-line.

    d. Prospective.

3. Bringing rapid medical care to the victim rather than bringing the victim to medical care is a basic principle of the—

    a. Triage system.

    b. Emergency medical services (EMS) system.

    c. First responder system.

    d. National Highway Traffic Safety Administration (NHTSA).

4. In an emergency, the first action of the citizen responder is to recognize that an emergency exists. Which is the second and most critical action?

    a. Providing care to the injured person

    b. Directing traffic around the scene

    c. Activating the EMS system by calling 9–1–1 or other local emergency number

    d. Taking the victim to the nearest emergency medical care facility

5. Which of the following workers may be a first responder?

    a. Police officer

    b. Industrial response team member

    c. Athletic trainer

    d. All of the above

6. Which person in the EMS system provides the transition between care given by the citizen responder and that provided by more advanced medical personnel?

    a. EMS dispatcher

    b. First responder

    c. Emergency medical technician

    d. Paramedic

7. When taking action at an emergency scene, one of your initial responsibilities is to—

    a. Determine any threats to the victim's life.

    b. Keep your skills and knowledge up to date.

    c. Record what you see, do, and hear at the scene.

    d. Transport the victim to a hospital.

8. Which statement best describes the emergency medical services (EMS) system?

    a. The EMS system provides an ambulance to transport the victim to the hospital.

    b. The EMS system consists of community resources organized to care for victims of sudden illness or injury.

    c. Personnel and equipment for removing victims from dangerous locations are part of the EMS system.

    d. The EMS system is organized to prevent the occurrence of injuries and sudden illness.

9. All of the following are components of an effective EMS system **except**—

    a. Regulation and policy.

    b. Communications.

    c. Human resources and training.

    d. Analysis.

10. Which link in the chain of survival has the goal of returning the injured or ill person to his or her previous state of health?

    a. First responder care

    b. Rehabilitation

    c. More advanced out-of-hospital care

    d. Hospital care

Notes

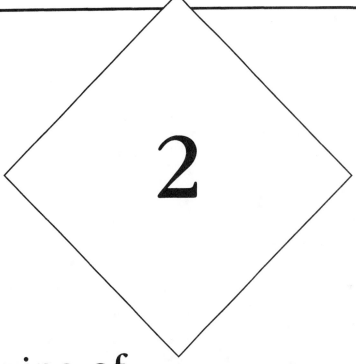

2

The Well-Being of the First Responder

◆ SUMMARY

An emotional crisis often results from an unexpected, shocking, and undesired event, such as the sudden loss of a loved one. Although people react differently in different situations, everyone experiences some or all of the stages of grief. By considering the nature of the incident, you can begin to prepare yourself to deal with its emotional aspects.

Regardless of the nature of the event, however, the care you provide to victims of any emotional crisis is very similar. Your care involves both appropriate verbal and non-verbal communication. It also requires you to understand that in some cases death is inevitable. In some situations, you may be overcome by emotion. Remember that self-help involves sharing your feelings with others.

Emergency scenes by their nature can be dangerous, so never approach a scene until you are sure it is safe. Your personal safety is always your first concern. Potential hazards at emergency scenes include traffic, fire, electricity, and hazardous materials. Other dangers include violence or crime scenes. If you have any doubt about the safety of a scene or if you are not trained and equipped to handle the situation, stay back and keep other untrained people out of the area. Be sure appropriate help has been called, and wait for properly trained and equipped personnel. Once you are sure the scene is safe, you will be expected to provide care to ill or injured victims.

◆ OUTLINE

Any items marked with ** indicate information found only in the Enrichment section of the text.

◆ LEARNING ACTIVITIES

Matching

Match each term with its definition. Write its letter on the line in front of the definition.

Terms

a. Assault

b. Cumulative stress

c. Emergency move

d. Emotional crisis

e. Critical Incident Stress Debriefing

Definitions

1. _____ A buildup of stress over a period of time

2. _____ An agitated state resulting from stress, often involving a significant event in a person's life

3. _____ Moving a victim before completing care when the victim is in immediate danger

4. _____ The threat of or actual abuse, either physical or sexual, resulting in injury and often emotional crisis

5. _____ A process by which emergency personnel are offered the support necessary to reduce emotional trauma associated with significant incidents

Matching

Terms

a. Physical assault

b. Rape

c. Active listening

d. Nonverbal communication

e. Suicide

Definitions

1. _____ A process that helps you more fully and accurately communicate with a victim

2. _____ A crime of violence, or one committed under threat of violence, involving a sexual attack

3. _____ Self-inflicted death

4. _____ Abuse that may result in injury to the body

5. _____ Conveying a message through body actions, such as assuming a nonthreatening posture

True/False

Circle T if the statement is true; circle F if it is false.

1. T F Stress is the body's normal response to any situation that changes a person's existing mental, physical, or emotional balance.

2. T F Individuals move from one grief stage to another in a predictable order.

3. T F Most emergency situations have little or no emotional impact on first responders.

4. T F A living will is a document that states that an individual does not wish to be resuscitated or further kept alive by mechanical means under certain circumstances.

5. T F The emotional impact of a critical incident varies based on the type of incident and number of victims rather than on the emotional makeup of the individuals involved.

6. T F A Critical Incident Stress Debriefing meeting is usually held within 72 to 96 hours of a major incident.

7. T F Response to a stressful situation differs from person to person.

8. T F A stage that involves blaming yourself for what happened is known as the disbelief stage.

9. T F In one way or another, a serious injury or sudden illness has an emotional impact on everyone involved.

**10. T F Once an earthquake is over, there are few risks for the inhabitants of the area.

11. T F You find a victim lying next to an overturned car. Gasoline is leaking from the area around the car near the victim. You should move the victim away from the car before providing emergency care.

12. T F An effective plan of action for an emergency response requires a large number of responders and vehicles.

**13. T F Emergency situations that a first responder might encounter include natural disasters, suicide, and fire.

14. T F Establishing a safety zone where all victims can be taken will ensure your safety at an emergency scene.

**15. T F Nonverbal communication includes the use of hand gestures, posture, facial expressions, and so on to convey a message.

**16. T F A victim of a sexual assault should be encouraged to shower after the incident.

**17. T F If trapped in a burning building, you should determine whether a door feels hot to the touch before opening it.

**18. T F If you are in a burning building, you should use the elevator if the elevator door feels cool to the touch.

**19. T F The first priority in a hostage situation is to gain access to any injured hostages to provide needed emergency care.

Short Answer

Read each statement or question and write the correct answer or answers in the space provided.

1. List three types of situations that will trigger a stress response.

2. List the six stages of the grieving process.

3. List five measures the first responder can use to help the victim and family deal with the dying process.

4. What types of situations might call for Critical Incident Stress Debriefing?

5. To ensure the safety of rescuers when approaching an emergency scene, a first responder must evaluate the scene for the following five elements. They are—

6. You are at the scene of a collision between a car and a tanker truck. You might perceive clues to the presence of hazardous materials. List at least five:

7. At the site of a motor vehicle crash, there are three situations in which you might park in a roadway to block traffic. They are—

8. Complete the table. Fill in the missing situation or the action you would take for the situation given.

Situation	Appropriate Action
a. Crime	
b. Wreckage	
**c. Suicide	

Situation	Appropriate Action
**d.	Do not enter structures that you suspect are unsafe. Call for trained and equipped personnel. Gather as much information as possible about the victim(s).
**e.	Report to the person in charge. Care for victims with the most life-threatening conditions first.

** 9. List five behaviors involved in active listening.

** 10. Identify six potential dangers to you, bystanders, and victims in the illustration.

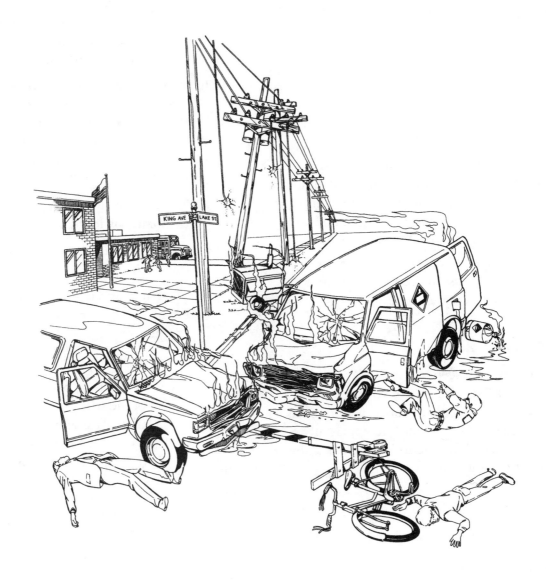

◆ CASE STUDIES

Read the case studies and answer the questions that follow.

**Case 2.1

You are called to the scene of a sexual assault. A 27-year-old woman is the victim. Upon arrival, you note that she is distraught, but quiet and controlled compared to her husband.

1. List at least six things you should do in caring for this victim.

2.   T   F   In this situation, you should separate the husband and wife as soon as possible to allow the husband to calm down and deal with his anger.

3.   T   F   The scene of this sexual assault should be treated as a crime scene.

**Case 2.2

You arrive at a scene where a truck has hit an electric utility pole. A high-voltage wire attached to the pole has broken and now is draped across the truck. Two apparently uninjured persons are still in the truck, and a crowd is gathering.

1. How far back from the scene should you move the bystanders?

   a. Half the distance between the two poles from which the broken wire had been strung.

   b. The distance between the two poles from which the broken wire had been strung.

   c. Twice the length of the span of the wire.

   d. The distance from the break in the wire to the closest power pole.

2.   T   F   You can safely move the wire off of the truck if you wear insulated gloves and use a dry stick or a nonmetal pole.

3. In sizing up the scene, you note a Department of Transportation-type placard on the rear door of the truck indicating the presence of hazardous materials. What information should you look for on the placard?

   a. The name or identifying number of the materials in the truck.

   b. The amount of chemicals usually in the truck.

   c. The name and telephone number of the manufacturer of the stored chemicals.

   d. All of the above.

4.   T   F   You should tell the occupants of the truck to get out of the truck carefully, as long as the wire is not sparking and they do not touch the wire.

◆ SELF-ASSESSMENT

Circle the letter of the best answer.

1. Techniques to help prevent "job burn-out" include—

   a. Changing lifestyles.

   b. Regular exercise.

   c. Balancing work, recreation, and family.

   d. All of the above.

2. Which stage of the grieving process involves the frustration of not being able to accept the event or a feeling that not enough was or is being done to help?

   a. Anger

   b. Anxiety

   c. Denial/disbelief

   d. Guilt/depression

3. One of the major reasons that emergency personnel experience emotional distress from their work is that—

   a. As they establish rapport with the victim, they become involved in the victim's pain and stress.

   b. They must avoid criticism, anger, or rejection of the victim's statements.

   c. Victims of an emotional crisis may be withdrawn or hysterical and entirely dependent on the emergency personnel for help.

   d. Frequently, there is no time to prepare mentally and emotionally for what will happen at the emergency scene.

4. Which of the following is the best example of an open-ended question?

   a. Are you having pain now?

   b. What problems are you having?

   c. Is the pain steady or does it come and go?

   d. Is there someone who can stay with you tonight?

5. Which stage of grief involves an unspoken promise of something in exchange for an extension of life or returning to the pre-event condition?

   a. Bargaining

   b. Anger

   c. Anxiety

   d. Acceptance

6. A written, legal expression of an individual's wishes regarding resuscitation and/or mechanical support is known as a—

   a. Last will and testament.

   b. DNR order.

   c. Living will.

   d. Debriefing.

7. Which of the following guidelines will help ensure your personal safety at an emergency scene?

   a. Take time to evaluate the scene before proceeding.

   b. Wear appropriate protective gear for the situation.

   c. Do not attempt activities for which you have not received the proper training.

   d. All of the above.

** 8. Why would you park in a roadway to block traffic?

   a. To stop all truck traffic

   b. To put out flares

   c. To identify the scene for more advanced medical personnel

   d. To protect rescuers

** 9. When approaching the scene of an automobile crash, you should—

   a. Carefully direct bystanders as to how to help find the victims.

   b. Move immediately to the victims who appear to be most seriously injured.

   c. Size up the overall situation before taking further action.

   d. Use your vehicle to slow down or stop traffic near the scene.

** 10. Which of the following is a behavior involved in active listening?

   a. Establishing physical contact with the victim

   b. Using a combination of open-ended and yes-no questions

   c. Contradicting statements from the victim that are obviously false

   d. Repeating back to the victim, in your own words, what he or she said

** 11. Which of the following is an example of nonverbal communication?

   a. Words of consolation

   b. Assuming a nonthreatening position

   c. Referral to a counseling center

   d. Having a bystander question the victim

** 12. A crime of violence that involves a sexual attack is known as—

   a. Arson.

   b. Battery.

   c. Assault.

   d. Rape.

** 13. In caring for a victim of a sexual assault you should—

   a. Cover the victim.

   b. Not disrupt the crime scene.

   c. Not question the victim about specifics of the crime.

   d. All of the above.

** 14. Which is your first concern when dealing with a victim of a physical assault?

   a. Your own safety

   b. The victim's physical injuries

   c. The victim's emotional state

   d. The emotional reactions of emergency care responders

** 15. Which of the following will give you the best chance to escape safely from a burning building?

   a. Stay upright as you run from the building.

   b. Cover your nose and mouth with a moist cloth.

   c. Stay close to the floor.

   d. a and b.

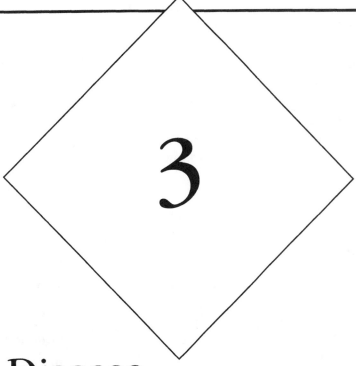

3

Preventing Disease Transmission

◆ SUMMARY

Although the body's immune system defends well against disease, pathogens can still enter the body and sometimes cause infection. These pathogens can be transmitted in four ways: by direct contact with an infected person; by indirect contact with a contaminated object; by inhaling air exhaled by an infected person; and through a bite from an infected animal, or insect.

Serious diseases include hepatitis, herpes, meningitis, tuberculosis, and HIV infection, including AIDS. You should know how the diseases are transmitted and take appropriate measures to protect yourself. Four conditions must be present for a disease to be transmitted.

The Occupational Safety and Health Administration (OSHA) has issued regulations on occupational exposure to bloodborne pathogens. The agency has determined that employees face a significant risk from occupational exposure to blood and other potentially infectious materials because they may contain bloodborne pathogens. OSHA concludes that this hazard can be minimized or eliminated using a combination of engineering and work practice controls, personal protective clothing and equipment, training, medical surveillance, hepatitis B vaccination, signs and labels, and other precautions. The OSHA regulations define the range of employees covered by the standard, and set forth specific requirements that employers must meet to maintain work sites in a clean and sanitary condition.

Following OSHA guidelines, especially the standard precautions or body substance isolation (BSI), greatly decreases your risk of contracting or transmitting an infectious disease. If you suspect that you have been exposed to such a disease, always document it, or notify your superior or *designated officer* and other involved personnel. Seek medical help and participate in any follow-up procedures.

Keep these principles concerning infectious disease in mind as you read the following chapters about providing care in specific situations. Even when you must act quickly, as in restoring breathing or circulation, take these precautions to reduce the risk of infection.

◆ OUTLINE

◆ LEARNING ACTIVITIES

Matching

Match each term with its definition. Write its letter on the line in front of the definition.

Terms

a. Antibody

b. Immunization

c. Hepatitis

d. Pathogen

e. Virus

f. Communicable disease

g. Body substance isolation

Definitions

1. _____ A substance introduced into the body to build resistance to a specific infection

2. _____ A disease-causing agent, also called a microorganism or germ

3. _____ A disease-causing agent that requires another organism to live and reproduce

4. _____ An infection-fighting protein released by white blood cells

5. _____ A condition that results in inflammation of the liver

6. _____ An infection control concept that approaches all body substances as potentially infectious

7. _____ Disease capable of being transmitted from people, animals, objects, and insects

True/False

Circle T if the statement is true; circle F if it is false.

1. T F HIV can be transmitted by casual contact, such as using a telephone or drinking fountain recently used by an infected person.

2. T F Vector-borne illnesses include rabies and Lyme disease.

3. T F If you think you have been exposed to an infectious disease while providing care, you should wait until the medical facility notifies you before taking any steps.

4. T F You should wear protective eyewear whenever you provide care to a bleeding victim.

5. T F For a disease to be transmitted from a victim to a rescuer, the victim must be infected with the disease.

6. T F Tuberculosis can be transmitted by contact with an infected person's urine or feces.

7. T F Despite its natural defenses, the body cannot always fight off infection.

8. T F Using plain soap and water to initially wash the visible soil from a vehicle floor and seats is dangerous because it could reactivate any HIV virus that might be in the dried blood on the floor.

9. T F Red blood cells are a basic component of the human immune system.

10. T F Direct contact transmission occurs when a person touches objects that have been contaminated by the blood or another body fluid of an infected person.

11. T F Personal protective equipment (PPE) includes equipment and supplies that prevent you from contacting infected materials.

12. T F Engineering controls are safeguards to isolate or remove the hazard from the workplace.

Short Answer

Read each statement or question and write the correct answer or answers in the space provided.

1. List the four conditions that must be present for a disease to be transmitted from one person to another.

2. If your equipment became contaminated with blood or other body fluids, what type of solution would you use to disinfect it?

3. Complete the table. Fill in the name(s) of the missing modes of transmission.

Disease	Mode of Transmission
HIV	
Tuberculosis	
Herpes	
Meningitis	
Hepatitis	

4. List six precautions you can take to prevent disease transmission.

◆ **CASE STUDIES**

Read the case studies and answer the questions that follow.

Case 3.1

You are called to a scene where a young boy has been bitten by a stray dog. The boy has two bleeding wounds on his leg. The bleeding is easily controlled by applying pressure to the wound.

1. The transmission of any infection from the dog to the victim is best described as—

   a. Direct contact transmission.

   b. Indirect contact transmission.

   c. Airborne transmission.

   d. Vector-borne transmission.

2. T F In caring for this victim and being exposed to his blood, you are at significant risk of infection for any diseases that might have been transmitted to the boy through the dog bite.

3. What disease might this dog transmit to the boy?

4. Which of the following protective items should you wear as you control the bleeding?

   a. Disposable gloves

   b. Protective eyewear

   c. Disposable mask

   d. All of the above

Case 3.2

While providing care for the victim of an assault, you suspect you have been exposed to an infectious disease.

1. The manner in which you report this exposure is often described in your

   _____ .

2. T F It is your responsibility to notify your superior and any necessary medical personnel immediately.

3. T   F   The OSHA regulations on bloodborne and airborne pathogens require employers to create an exposure control plan and provide employee training relative to these regulations

◆ SELF-ASSESSMENT

Circle the letter of the best answer.

1. Pathogens that depend on another living organism to live and reproduce are—

    a. Bacteria.

    b. Protozoa.

    c. Viruses.

    d. Fungi.

2. Disease transmission from a victim to a first responder requires four conditions. Which of the following is a condition?

    a. The victim requiring care must be infected with the disease.

    b. The first responder providing care must be exposed to the infected victim's body fluids.

    c. There must be enough of the pathogen present to cause infection.

    d. All of the above.

3. Basic components of the immune system are—

    a. Red blood cells.

    b. White blood cells.

    c. Platelets.

    d. Serum.

4. Through which route is herpes transmitted?

    a. Direct contact

    b. Indirect contact

    c. Airborne transmission

    d. All of the above

5. Which of the following protective equipment should a first responder wear to prevent disease transmission when handling and cleaning equipment contaminated with blood?

    a. Protective eyewear

    b. Disposable mask

    c. Disposable gloves

    d. All of the above

6. How much household chlorine bleach is needed in a gallon of water to produce an effective solution for disinfecting equipment such as splints and stethoscopes?

    a. 1 pint

    b. 1 cup

    c. $1/2$ cup

    d. $1/4$ cup

7. You think you have been exposed to an infectious disease while providing care. You would first—

    a. Try to find out which disease it was.

    b. Notify your superior and any involved medical personnel.

    c. Go to be tested at a hospital.

    d. All of the above.

8. In which of the following ways can a pathogen enter the body?

   a. Direct contact transmission

   b. Indirect contact transmission

   c. Airborne transmission

   d. All of the above

9. Jaundice is a condition caused by illness affecting the—

   a. Liver.

   b. Heart.

   c. Brain.

   d. Spleen.

10. The infectious disease most likely to be transmitted by contaminated shellfish is—

    a. Tuberculosis.

    b. Meningitis.

    c. Hepatitis A.

    d. Chlamydia.

11. Employers must ensure that medical evaluations, procedures, and post-exposure evaluation and follow-up care are—

    a. Made available to employees for a fee.

    b. Provided under the supervision of an EMT.

    c. Made available to employees at a time and date specified by the employer.

    d. Provided according to the current recommendations of the U.S. Public Health Service.

Notes

PRACTICE SESSION: *Removing Gloves*

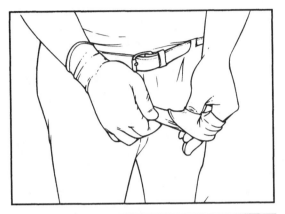

☐ **Partially remove first glove**

- ◆ Pinch glove at the wrist, being careful to touch only the glove's outside surface.
- ◆ Pull glove towards the fingertips without completely removing it.
- ◆ The glove is now inside out.

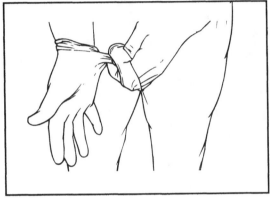

☐ **Remove second glove**

- ◆ With partially gloved hand, pinch the exterior of second glove.

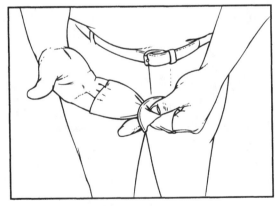

☐ ◆ Pull the second glove toward the fingertips until it is inside out, then remove it completely.

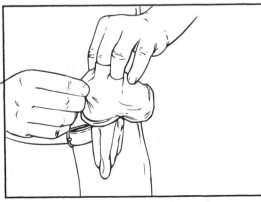

☐ **Finish removing both gloves**

- ◆ Grasp both gloves with your free hand.
- ◆ Touch only the clean interior surface of the glove.

After removing both gloves...

- ◆ Discard gloves in an appropriate container.
- ◆ Wash your hands thoroughly.

Notes

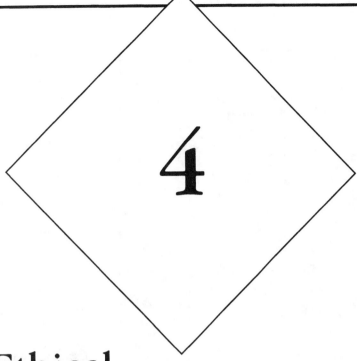

Legal and Ethical Issues

◆ SUMMARY

In your role as an emergency care provider, you are guided by certain legal parameters, such as the duty to act and professional standards of care. Victims of injury or illness have a right to expect competent initial care by a first responder. Part of a first responder's responsibility lies not only in giving competent care, but also in keeping up skills and knowledge through refresher programs and continuing education.

Regardless of your profession, when you are called to help a victim of injury or sudden illness, you assume the role of an emergency care provider. When an emergency occurs, the people in your care, as well as assisting bystanders, will expect you to know what to do. Be prepared to think and act accordingly. What to do, however, often involves more than giving emergency care.

Keeping information that you learn about a victim confidential is very important. The information that you learn as you give care can directly affect the outcome of the victim's condition. Victims could lose trust in first responders who do not protect their confidentiality. Effective documentation is important in maintaining the standard of care for a victim and may provide legal protection for you and the organization you represent.

◆ OUTLINE

Any items marked with ** indicate information found only in the Enrichment section of the text.

◆LEARNING ACTIVITIES

Matching

Match each term with its definition. Write its letter on the line in front of the definition.

Terms

a. Abandonment

b. Confidentiality

c. Consent

d. Duty to Act

e. Good Samaritan laws

f. Negligence

g. Refusal of care

h. Scope of practice

i. Standard of care

Definitions

1. _____ Failure to provide the appropriate level of care, which leads to injury of or damage to a victim

2. _____ Permission to provide care, given by an ill or injured person

3. _____ Ending the care of an ill or injured person without obtaining that person's consent

4. _____ A legal responsibility of some individuals to provide a reasonable standard of emergency care

5. _____ The criterion established for the extent and quality of a first responder's care

6. _____ The declining of care by a competent person

7. _____ Laws that protect people who willingly give emergency care without accepting anything in return

8. _____ The range of duties and skills a first responder is allowed and expected to perform when necessary

9. _____ Protecting a victim's privacy by not revealing any personal information you learn about the victim

**Matching

Match each term with its definition. Write its letter on the line in front of the definition.

Terms

a. Developmentally disabled

b. Hearing impaired

c. Visually impaired

d. Physically disabled

Definitions

1. _____ A person who is either blind or partially blind

2. _____ A person with impaired mental function resulting from injury or genetics

3. _____ A person who is born with or acquires a disability that interferes with normal movement and activity

4. _____ A person who is deaf or partially deaf

True/False

Circle T if the statement is true; circle F if it is false.

1. T F First responders are frequently sued for their actions in providing emergency care.

2. T F The range of duties and skills a first responder is allowed and expected to perform when necessary is called the standard of care.

3. T F As a first responder, you have an ethical obligation to carry out your duties and responsibilities in a professional manner.

4. T F Advance directives and Do Not Resuscitate (DNR) Orders are usually written for people who are over 75 years of age.

5. T F If you are called to give care to a victim of violence or crime and law enforcement personnel are not present, you should notify them.

6. T F Abuse is the legal term used to describe the unlawful touching of a victim without the victim's consent.

7. T F A person could be negligent either by acting wrongly or failing to act at all.

8. T F A competent, conscious adult has the right to refuse care even if he or she is obviously seriously injured.

9. T F If a lawyer is present at the scene of an accident, it is appropriate to discuss victim information with him or her if you think someone may be sued.

**10. T F The assessment of a visually impaired victim should be very similar to the assessment of a victim who is not visually impaired.

**11. T F The main reasons for the increased risk of serious head injuries in the elderly are increasingly poor eyesight and, more frequently, loss of balance.

**12.   T   F   When caring for a person with a physical disability who is injured, you should care for any problems you detect that could be related to the injury as if they are new rather than preexisting.

**13.   T   F   A person who is termed developmentally disabled must be physically challenged.

**14.   T   F   When providing care for an elderly victim, you should not waste time determining whether any confusion is the result of injury or a preexisting condition.

**15.   T   F   One of the problems you may face in caring for a developmentally disabled person is the victim's anxiety and fear resulting from disruption of his or her otherwise orderly life.

**16.   T   F   You will often have to speak a bit louder and more slowly than usual to effectively communicate with a person who is visually impaired.

Short Answer

Read each statement or question and write the correct answer or answers in the space provided.

1. Explain the following terms: expressed consent; implied consent.

2. List the four components that must be present for a lawsuit charging negligence to be successful.

** 3. List four general types of mentally and physically disabled victims.

◆ CASE STUDIES

Read the case studies and answer the following questions.

Case 4.1

While you are returning home one evening from work, the car in front of you suddenly crosses the center line and crashes into an embankment on the opposite side of the road. As you pull up next to the car, you notice that the driver is slumped across the steering wheel and is not moving.

1. In this situation, do you have a duty to act? If so, why?

2. If you decide to act in this situation, your first concern should be to—

   a. Determine threats to the victim.

   b. Summon advanced medical personnel as needed.

   c. Provide care for the victim(s).

   d. Ensure safety for yourself and any bystanders.

3. What potential dangers to you and any bystanders at the scene may be present?

4. T F After the victim has been cared for, you should discuss the care you gave and any information you learned about the victim with lawyers and reporters.

**Case 4.2

You are summoned to the home of a 76-year-old woman. When you arrive, a neighbor tells you she found her lying on her bathroom floor, conscious, but unable to get up. The victim does not recognize her neighbor and cannot remember what happened. She complains of pain in her left leg and hip. Her pulse and breathing seem normal, and she is able to converse with you. You ask her what day it is, and she answers incorrectly.

1. T F In caring for this woman, you should ask about and look for any medications she has been taking in the past few days.

2. In what way would you talk with this woman to determine if there are any other problems she may have?

   a. Look at her and talk loudly so she can hear you.

   b. Stand at her side and talk into her ear.

   c. Get at eye level so she can see and hear you.

   d. Stand above her and talk to her.

**Case 4.3

A man has fallen on an icy sidewalk and appears to have broken his left forearm. He is conscious and breathing. You introduce yourself and ask him what happened. He does not answer you, but shakes his head "No" and points to his ear.

1. List three ways in which you might be able to communicate more effectively with this victim.

2. T F Because of the victim's condition, you will have to assume that he cannot speak. You will need to rely on your physical assessment and information from bystanders to determine the appropriate treatment.

◆ SELF-ASSESSMENT

Circle the letter of the best answer.

1. A legal responsibility of some individuals to provide a reasonable standard of emergency care is called—

   a. Standard of practice.

   b. Duty to act.

   c. Standard of care.

   d. Paraprofessional duty.

2. The criterion established that includes the extent and quality of a first responder's care is called—

   a. Scope of practice.

   b. Duty to act.

   c. Standard of care.

   d. Paraprofessional duty.

3. Laws that protect people who willingly give emergency care without accepting anything in return are called—

   a. Citizen Responder laws.

   b. Hold Harmless laws.

   c. Good Samaritan laws.

   d. Medical Immunity laws.

4. Unless an illness or injury is life threatening, in order for a first responder to be able to provide care to a child, he or she must first obtain permission from a parent or guardian. This permission is called—

   a. Implied consent.

   b. Minor's consent.

   c. Expressed consent.

   d. Informed consent.

5. Ending care of an ill or injured person without that person's consent or without ensuring that someone with equal or greater training will continue that care is called—

   a. Consent.

   b. Good Samaritan laws.

   c. Refusal of care.

   d. Abandonment.

6. All of the following statements about documentation are correct except—

   a. Documenting your care is nearly as important as the care itself.

   b. Your record will help advanced healthcare professionals assess the victim and continue care.

   c. Documentation laws are established by the EMS agency.

   d. Your record is a legal document and is important if legal action occurs.

7. Carrying out your duties and responsibilities in a professional manner is an example of a/an—

   a. Ethical responsibility.

   b. Duty to act.

   c. Issue of confidentiality.

   d. Scope of practice.

** 8. Which of the following actions will help you effectively assess an elderly person?

   a. Getting in a position above the victim

   b. Carefully explaining what you wish to do

   c. Placing the victim in a sitting position

   d. Asking questions only of the elderly person

** 9. Which of the following should you do in moving a person with a visual impairment who can walk?

    a. Walk slowly behind him or her with your hand on their back.

    b. Walk beside the victim, and let him or her grasp your arm while you are walking.

    c. Grasp the victim's arm or belt, and support the victim as you walk.

    d. Walk in front of the victim, and have him or her keep a hand on your shoulder.

** 10. To effectively communicate with a hearing-impaired person who reads lips, you must remember to—

    a. Look at the victim when you speak.

    b. Divide your words into syllables and pronounce them one at a time.

    c. Make certain you are in a position in which the person can see you clearly.

    d. a and c.

Notes

Notes

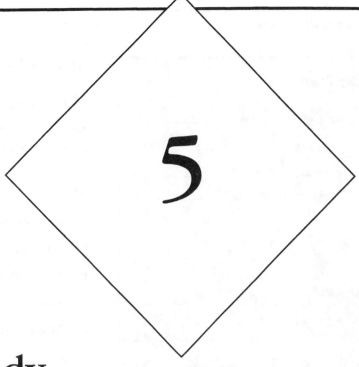

Human Body
Systems

◆ SUMMARY

The body includes a number of body systems, all of which must work together for the body to function properly. The brain, the center of the nervous system, controls all body functions, including those of the other body systems. Knowing a few key structures, their functions, and their locations helps you understand more about these body systems.

◆ OUTLINE

Any items marked with ** indicate information found only in the Enrichment section of the text.

◆ LEARNING ACTIVITIES

Matching

Match each term with its definition. Write its letter on the line in front of the definition.

Terms

a. Nervous System

b. Integumentary system

c. Musculoskeletal system

d. Tissue

e. Respiratory system

Definitions

1. _____ A collection of similar cells that performs a specific function

2. _____ A body system that activates, coordinates, and controls the activity of all body systems

3. _____ A body system responsible for supporting the body, allowing movement, and protecting internal organs

4. _____ A body system consisting of the skin, hair, and nails

5. _____ A group of organs and other structures that brings air into the body and removes waste products

**Matching

Match each term with its definition. Write its letter on the line in front of the definition.

Terms

a. Genitourinary system

b. Endocrine system

c. Lateral

d. Inferior

e. Distal

Definitions

1. _____ A body system that regulates and coordinates the activities of other body systems by producing chemicals that influence the activity of tissues

2. _____ Farthest from the center or midline

3. _____ A body system that eliminates wastes and enables reproduction

4. _____ Points away from the trunk

5. _____ Lower; below in relation to another structure

True/False

Circle T if the statement is true; circle F if it is false.

1. T   F   For the body to maintain a consistently healthy state, body systems must function independently.

2. T   F   The cranial cavity contains the spinal cord and the nerves.

3. T   F   The exchange of oxygen and carbon dioxide occurs in the alveoli.

4. T   F   Although respiratory arrest is a serious problem, it is not usually life threatening.

5. T   F   The musculoskeletal system stores minerals and produces blood cells.

6. T   F   The primary waste gas expelled during exhalation is carbon dioxide.

7. T   F   Injuries to the musculoskeletal system may result in life-threatening damage to the circulatory and respiratory systems.

8. T   F   The nervous and circulatory systems coordinate and regulate all body functions.

9. T   F   The heart, blood, and blood vessels are major components of the circulatory system.

10. T   F   Injuries to the nervous system may result in impairment of the integumentary system.

**11. T   F   Most digestive system organs are protected by the skeletal system.

**12. T   F   Glands are organs that release fluid into the blood or onto the skin.

Short Answer

Read each statement or question and write the correct answer or answers in the space provided.

** 1. Identify each body cavity.

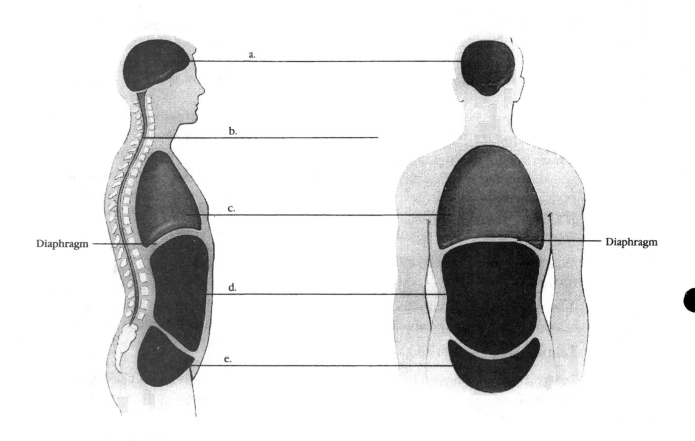

** 2. List the major structures in the body cavities.

a. _____

b. _____

c. _____

d. _____

3. Identify the structures of the respiratory system.

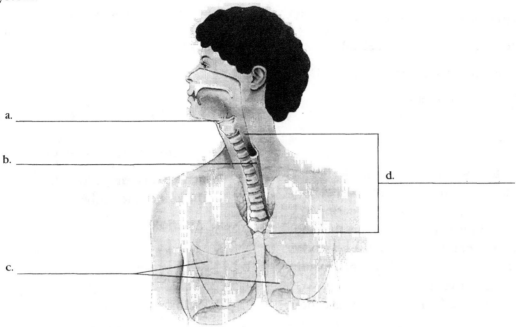

a. _____

b. _____

d. _____

c. _____

** 4. Describe the body in the "anatomical position."

◆ CASE STUDIES

Read the case studies and answer the questions that follow.

Case 5.1

While mowing her lawn, a woman runs over a piece of fence wire. The piece of wire is propelled backwards and makes a deep laceration on her lower leg.

** 1. Using correct medical terminology, describe the location of her injury in relation to these other body structures:

Knee: _____

Ankle: _____

** 2. Is the injury anterior or posterior?

** 3. Is the injury on the medial or lateral side of the leg?

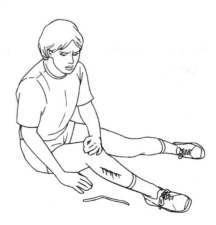

4. Which two body systems will interact initially to alert the victim to this injury?

   a. Circulatory, respiratory

   b. Respiratory, musculoskeletal

   c. Integumentary, nervous

   d. Nervous, respiratory

**Case 5.2

Late one afternoon a woman faints in her office. You are summoned to the scene. As you examine her, you see she is wearing a medical-alert bracelet that indicates that she is an insulin-dependent diabetic. A co-worker tells you that the woman did take her insulin today but has not yet eaten and twenty minutes ago worked out in the fitness center.

1. Diabetes is a condition that results from a problem in which system?

   a. Circulatory

   b. Integumentary

   c. Endocrine

   d. Nervous

2. T   F   Most serious illnesses caused by malfunctions of this system develop slowly.

3. What kind of organs make up this system?

4. What is the primary function of these organs?

5. Many of these organs release their substances into the circulatory system to influence tissue activity in various parts of the body. What are these substances called?

◆ SELF-ASSESSMENT

Circle the letter of the best answer.

1. Which vessels carry blood from the heart to the rest of the body?

   a. Arterioles

   b. Arteries

   c. Venules

   d. Veins

2. In reaction to cold, the skin becomes pale and shows what is called "goose-flesh." Which two systems are interacting with the skin to maintain body temperature?

   a. Nervous, musculoskeletal

   b. Respiratory, integumentary

   c. Circulatory, musculoskeletal

   d   Nervous, circulatory

3. The three primary functions of the nervous system are—

   a. Sensory, motor, integrated.

   b. Consciousness, memory, emotions.

   c. Visual, olfactory, auditory.

   d. Consciousness, regulation, language.

4. Which structure in the airway prevents liquids and solids from entering the lungs?

   a. Epiglottis

   b. Uvula

   c. Trachea

   d. Esophagus

5. One of the main functions of the integumentary system is to—

    a. Transmit information to the brain.

    b. Produce blood cells.

    c. Prevent infection.

    d. Secrete hormones.

6. Which structure is not part of the thoracic cavity?

    a. Liver

    b. Heart

    c. Lungs

    d. Rib cage

7. The two body systems that work together to provide oxygen for the cells of the body are—

    a. Musculoskeletal and integumentary.

    b. Respiratory and circulatory.

    c. Integumentary and respiratory.

    d. Circulatory and musculoskeletal.

8. Transporting nutrients and oxygen to body cells and removing waste products are functions of the—

    a. Circulatory system.

    b. Respiratory system.

    c. Digestive system.

    d. Endocrine system.

* * 9. A person in the anatomical position is standing—

    a. Arms out, palms facing downward.

    b. Arms at the side, palms facing backward.

    c. Arms out, palms facing forward.

    d. Arms at the side, palms facing forward.

* *10. In comparison to the elbow, the shoulder is described as ____, whereas the hand is _____ .

    a. Inferior, superior

    b. Proximal, distal

    c. Superior, inferior

    d. Distal, proximal

Notes

Notes

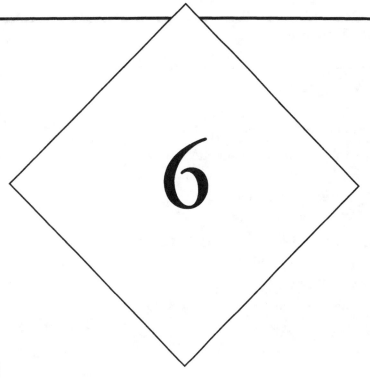

6

Lifting and Moving

◆ SUMMARY

Take the time to survey the scene and determine if moving the victim is absolutely necessary before attempting to give care. Remember that your safety, and the safety of your partner, always comes first. This is especially true in incidents involving hazardous materials.

Avoid the common mistake of forcibly moving an ill or injured person unnecessarily. If you recognize a potentially life-threatening situation that requires the victim to be moved immediately, use one of the techniques described in this chapter. Use the safest and easiest method to rapidly move the victim without causing injury to either yourself or the victim.

It is important for you to familiarize yourself with some of the typical equipment used in the local EMS systems. You should practice using the different types of stretchers and backboards, as you could be called on to assist the EMS providers in your area.

◆ LEARNING ACTIVITIES

Matching

Match each term with its definition. Write its letter on the line in front of the definition.

Terms

a. Fire fighter's carry

b. Pack-strap carry

c. Clothes drag

d. Shoulder drag

e. Direct lift

Definitions

1. _____ A method to move a victim by reaching under the victim's armpits (from the back), grasping the victim's forearms, and dragging the victim to safety

2. _____ A method of quickly moving a victim to safety that can be performed by one rescuer and allows you to have one of your hands free

3. _____ A method of moving a victim that uses three rescuers

4. _____ An appropriate move for a person suspected of having a head or spine injury

5. _____ A move that is made by positioning yourself with your back to the victim so that your shoulders fit into the victim's armpits; cross the victim's arms in front of you and lift the victim

True/False

Circle T if the statement is true; circle F if it is false.

1. T F   You should move a victim before providing emergency care if the victim is found in an uncomfortable position.

2. T F   The pack-strap carry can be used on both conscious and unconscious victims.

3. T F   The walking assist is the most basic move that requires the assistance of two rescuers.

4. T F   As a general rule, to ensure a victim's safety, you should face forward and move carefully forward when moving a victim.

5. T F   Body mechanics refers to the field of physiology that studies muscular actions and the function of the muscles in maintaining the posture of the body.

6. T F   An advantage of the fire fighter's carry is that it leaves one of the rescuer's hands free.

7. T F   An unresponsive victim without trauma should be placed in the recovery position by rolling the victim onto his or her side.

8. T F The size of the victim should not be a consideration when performing a rescue move.

9. T F Using the pack-strap carry with an unconscious victim requires two rescuers.

10. T F When moving a victim, walk carefully by taking short steps.

Short Answer

Read each statement or question and write the correct answer or answers in the space provided.

1. What are the three general situations in which you may need to move a victim before providing emergency care?

2. List five safety precautions the first responder should consider before moving the victim.

3. What three general considerations require the rescuer to perform an emergency move?

4. What are the three most common types of moves used by first responders?

◆ CASE STUDY

Read the case studies and answer the questions that follow.

Case 6.1

You are called to an apartment building where a middle-aged woman has fallen down a flight of stairs while trying to escape from a fire. She is lying at the base of the steps. The fire is spreading, and the stairwell is filling with smoke. You can see on approaching her that she has a laceration on her forehead and a marked deformity of her left leg. She does not respond when you speak to her.

1. What five factors would you take into consideration before moving the victim?

2. Which of the following techniques would be appropriate for you as a single rescuer to use to move this victim out of the building?

   a. Walking assist

   b. Pack-strap carry

   c. Clothes drag

   d. Foot drag

◆ SELF-ASSESSMENT

Circle the letter of the best answer.

1. How can you protect yourself from injury when moving a victim?

   a. Lift with your legs and back.

   b. Bend your body at the knees and hips.

   c. Walk slowly backward rather than forward.

   d. Use strides as long as you can comfortably take.

2. A victim has jumped from the second story of a burning building and is lying on the ground just below the fire. She has a laceration on her thigh and is barely conscious. You decide you must move her before providing emergency care. A second rescuer is with you. Which would be the most appropriate emergency move for you to use with this victim?

   a. Walking assist

   b. Seat carry

   c. Fire fighter's carry

   d. Clothes drag

3. Guidelines you should follow to protect yourself and the victim when moving someone include which of the following?

   a. Only attempt to move a victim you are sure you can safely and comfortably handle.

   b. Communicate clearly and frequently with your partner, the victim, and other EMS providers.

   c. Avoid bending or twisting a victim with a possible head, neck, or back injury.

   d. All of the above.

4. Which of the following moves can be done by a single rescuer?

   a. Direct lift

   b. Draw sheet move

   c. Fire fighter's carry

   d. Direct carry

5. In this moving technique, one rescuer kneels behind the victim keeping his or her back straight and reaches under the victim's arms and grasps the victim's opposite wrists. The second rescuer kneels between the victim's legs and firmly grasps around the knees and thighs. On a signal from the rescuer at the victim's head, both rescuers move from a crouching position to a standing position. This method of moving a victim is called—

   a. Extremity lift

   b. Pack-strap carry

   c. Direct carry

   d. Direct lift

6. To place a victim in the fire fighter's carry, the victim must first be—

   a. Supported and standing next to you.

   b. Brought to a sitting position.

   c. Lying on his or her back beside you.

   d. On one side, arms extended over the head.

7. In which of the following situations would you move a victim before providing emergency care?

   a. The victim is lying unconscious on a sidewalk, and a large crowd of bystanders has gathered.

   b. The victim is sitting in a truck on the shoulder of a busy highway and is complaining of chest pain.

   c. The victim is sitting in his car in a supermarket parking lot and has no pulse and is not breathing.

   d. The victim has collapsed unconscious in the doorway of an office building and is blocking the doorway.

8. The most basic of all the moves is the—

    a. Clothes drag.

    b. Walking assist.

    c. Direct carry.

    d. Extremity lift.

9. Some of the most commonly used transport devices that you will see as a first responder include all of the following except—

    a. Ambulance cots.

    b. Stair chairs.

    c. Long backboards.

    d. Wheel chairs.

10. Which of the following terms describes the field of physiology that studies muscular actions and the function of the muscles in maintaining the posture of the body.

    a. Lifting techniques

    b. Lifting mechanics

    c. Body mechanics

    d. Body techniques

Notes

Notes

PRACTICE SESSION: *Walking Assist (One or Two Rescuers)*

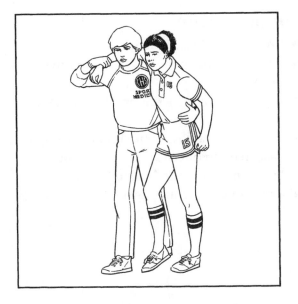

☐ **Support victim**
- ◆ Place victim's arm across your shoulder.
- ◆ Hold the arm with one hand.
- ◆ Place your other hand around victim's waist.

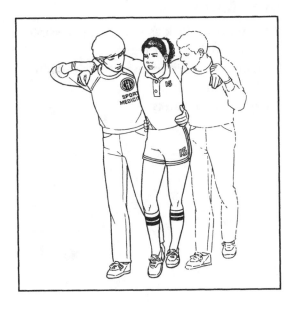

☐ **Move victim**
- ◆ Support victim's weight while you walk.
- ◆ If second rescuer is present, second rescuer supports victim in same way from other side.
- ◆ Walk victim to safety.

PRACTICE SESSION: *Fire Fighter's Carry*

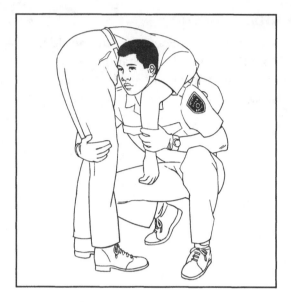

☐ Support victim

- ◆ Kneel down beside victim.
- ◆ Support victim in a seated or standing position facing you.
- ◆ If possible, have victim or a bystander help you.
- ◆ Hoist victim across your shoulders lengthwise, feet on one side, head on other.
- ◆ Put your arm around victim's legs.
- ◆ Grasp one of victim's arms.

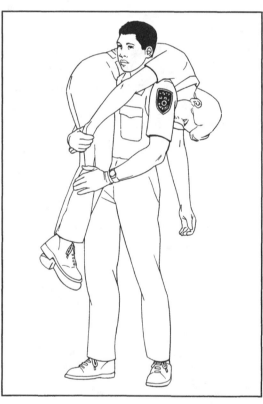

☐ Move victim

- ◆ Keeping your back as straight as possible, stand up, using your legs.
- ◆ Transfer your grip from victim's thigh to victim's arm.
- ◆ Carry victim to safety.

PRACTICE SESSION: *Pack-Strap Carry*

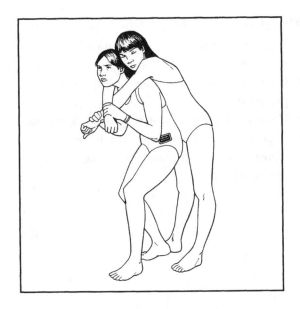

☐ **Support victim**

- ◆ Support victim in standing position.
- ◆ If possible, have victim or a bystander help you.
- ◆ Position yourself with back to victim, knees bent, so that your shoulders fit into victim's armpits.
- ◆ Cross victim's arms in front of you. Grasp victim's wrists.

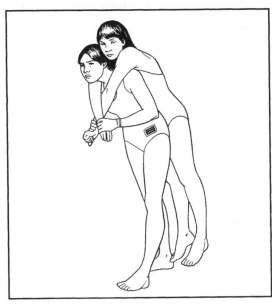

☐ **Move victim**

- ◆ Lean forward and pull victim up onto your back.
- ◆ Keeping your back as straight as possible, stand up, using your legs.
- ◆ Carry victim to safety.
- ◆ If possible, hold both of victim's wrists with one hand to free other hand to open doors and remove obstructions.

PRACTICE SESSION: *Two-Person Seat Carry*

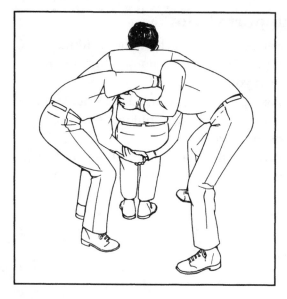

☐ **Support victim**

- ◆ Support victim in seated or standing position.
- ◆ Have victim or bystander help you, if possible.
- ◆ Place victim's arm around rescuers' necks.
- ◆ Each rescuer places one arm across victim's back and places other arm under victim's thighs.

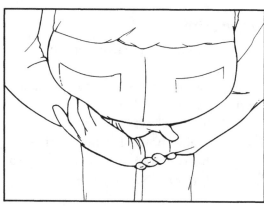

- ◆ Interlock forearms and wrists behind the victim's legs.

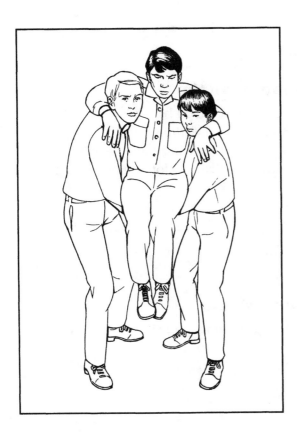

□ **Move victim**

◆ Lift victim in seat formed by rescuers' arms.

◆ Lift using your legs not your back.

◆ Carry victim to safety.

PRACTICE SESSION: *Clothes Drag*

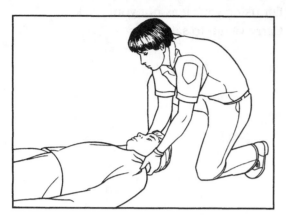

☐ **Support victim**

♦ Position victim on back.
♦ Kneel behind victim's head.
♦ Support victim's head and neck by gathering victim's clothing behind neck.

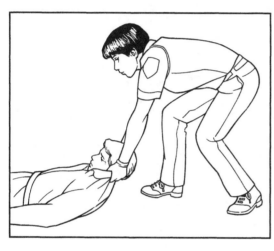

☐ **Move victim**

♦ Using clothing, pull victim to safety.

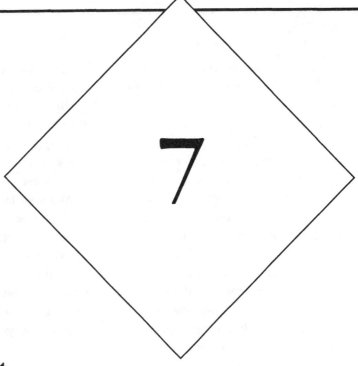

Assessment

◆ **SUMMARY**

When you respond to an emergency, guide your actions by following a standardized plan. This plan reminds you of what to do and when to do it. It helps ensure your safety and the safety of others. It also helps ensure that necessary or urgent care is provided for life-threatening emergencies.

First, size up the scene. Make sure there are no dangers to you, the victim, and bystanders. Consider the mechanism of injury or nature of illness.

Second, perform an initial assessment. Check consciousness, airway, breathing, and circulation. Determine if there are any immediate threats to life, such as the absence of breathing or pulse, or the presence of severe external bleeding.

Third, perform a physical exam to find and care for any other problems that are not an immediate threat to life but might become serious if you do not recognize them and provide care. This "head-to-toe" physical exam involves looking at and feeling the body for abnormalities. Use the mnemonic DOTS (**D**eformity, **O**pen injuries, **T**enderness, **S**welling) as you perform the physical exam.

Fourth, obtain pertinent history from the victim. This is especially important if the victim is suffering from an illness that has already been diagnosed and is being cared for by a physician. Whether you obtain the history before, after, or during the physical exam does not matter. Use the mnemonic SAMPLE (**S**igns and symptoms, **A**llergies, **M**edications, **P**ertinent past history, **L**ast oral intake, **E**vents leading up to the incident) to gather all of the necessary information.

Fifth, perform an ongoing assessment until more advanced personnel arrive and take over.

Repeat the initial assessment every 5 minutes for unstable victims and every 15 minutes for stable ones. Repeat the physical exam and history as needed.

Although this plan of action can help you decide what care to give in any emergency, providing care is not an exact science. Because each emergency and each victim is unique, an emergency may not occur exactly as it did in a classroom setting. Even within a single emergency, the care needed may change from one moment to the next. For example, the initial assessment may indicate the victim is conscious, breathing, has a pulse, and has no severe bleeding. However, during your physical exam, you may notice that the victim begins to experience breathing difficulty. At this point, there is a need to summon more advanced medical personnel, if this has not already been done, and provide appropriate care. Provide necessary information about the victim's condition once these personnel arrive.

Many variables exist when dealing with emergencies. You do not need to "diagnose" what is wrong with the victim to provide appropriate care. Use this plan of action as a guideline to help you assess any victim's condition. Always remember the steps of this plan. They form the basis for providing care in any emergency.

◆ OUTLINE

Any items marked with ** indicate information found only in the Enrichment section of the text.

◆ LEARNING ACTIVITIES

Matching

Match each term with its definition. Write its letter on the line in front of the definition.

Terms

a. Physical exam

b. Initial assessment

c. Vital signs

d. Ongoing assessment

e. Symptom

f. Level of consciousness

Definitions

1. _____ Something the victim tells you about his or her condition

2. _____ A check for conditions that are an immediate threat to life

3. _____ Examination performed immediately after the initial assessment

4. _____ A person's state of awareness or mental status

5. _____ Repeating the initial assessment and physical exam while awaiting the arrival of EMS personnel

6. _____ Information obtained by checking consciousness, breathing, pulse, and skin

**Matching

Match each term with its definition. Write its letter on the line in front of the definition.

Terms

a. Systolic blood pressure

b. Auscultation

c. Ventricles

d. Diastolic blood pressure

e. Palpation

Definitions

1. _____ The act of feeling an area of the body, such as the radial artery in the wrist

2. _____ The process of listening to sounds with a stethoscope

3. _____ The pressure in the arteries during the heart's working phase

4. _____ The pressure in the arteries during the heart's resting phase

5. _____ The lower two chambers of the heart

True/False

Circle T if the statement is true; circle F if it is false.

1. T F In the initial assessment, checking circulation includes checking for a pulse, severe bleeding, and possible broken bones.

2. T F You are summoned to a scene where a woman is complaining of pain in her hip. She states that it gets worse when she stands up and moves around, but lets up if she rests. This victim is experiencing an immediately life-threatening problem.

3. T F The physical exam is intended to find life-threatening problems not discovered in the initial assessment.

4. T F By rechecking vital signs, you will be able to discover changes in a victim's condition over time.

5. T F When performing the physical examination, you should ask the victim to carefully move any body part in which there is pain.

6. T F The mnemonic AVPU is used to reflect a victim's level of consciousness.

7. T F A victim who is "alert" cannot be disoriented.

8. T F Before providing care for any victim, you should make sure the scene is safe for the victim and rescuers.

9. T F The first thing you should do at any emergency scene is check victims for life-threatening injuries.

10. T F If you determine that a scene is dangerous and you cannot reach a victim, you should call more advanced medical personnel and attempt to keep bystanders from becoming additional victims.

11. T F You should perform an initial assessment on every victim because it allows you to identify conditions that threaten the victim's life.

12. T F When you ask, "Are you O.K.?," a victim who can answer this question is conscious, breathing, and has a pulse.

13. T F Forming a general impression of the victim's condition is done during the physical exam.

14. T F The mechanism of injury often provides clues as to how the incident occurred and the possible extent of injury to the victim.

15. T F Signs are what the victim tells you about his or her condition.

**16. T F Systolic blood pressure is the pressure in the arteries when the heart is at rest and refilling.

**17. T F Auscultation is the process of using a stethoscope and blood pressure cuff to listen for characteristic blood pressure sounds.

Short Answer

Read each statement or question and write the correct answer or answers in the space provided.

1. What are the five steps of the emergency plan of action?

2. What are the four components to consider during scene size-up?

3. What are the three components of the initial assessment?

4. What do the letters AVPU stand for in regard to a victim's level of consciousness?

5. What is the purpose of the physical exam?

6. What does the SAMPLE history include?

** 7. What equipment allows you to measure blood pressure by auscultation?

** 8. How would you write a blood pressure that was 70 millimeters of mercury (mm Hg) diastolic and 110 mm Hg systolic?

◆ CASE STUDIES

Read the case studies below and answer the questions that follow.

Case 7.1

You are summoned to the university swimming pool to care for an injured swimmer. You find a 21-year-old man lying beside the pool, not moving. You are unable to arouse him. You confirm that he is breathing and has a pulse.

1. What should you do next?

    a. Check his pupils.

    b. Do a physical exam.

    c. Look for severe bleeding.

    d. Help the victim to his feet.

2. Assuming more advanced medical personnel have been summoned, what should you do next?

    a. Cover him with a blanket to prevent heat loss.

    b. Maintain an open airway.

    c. Request a medical history from the office.

    d. Perform a physical exam.

3. The victim's vital signs are assessed and found as listed below. Place a check in front of those that are abnormal findings.

    ____ Pulse: 70 and regular

    ____ Respirations: 14

    ____ Blood pressure: 190/105

    ____ Level of consciousness: Unable to respond to questions

Case 7.2

You are called to a scene where a 13-year-old boy has fallen out of a tree. When you arrive, he is lying on the ground crying and holding his left arm. He appears to be very upset and wants to get up.

1. In which circumstance should you move this victim before providing care?

    a. When the victim is complaining of being in an uncomfortable position

    b. When it is impossible to splint fractures or bandage wounds without moving the victim

    c. When the victim is situated so that more advanced medical personnel will have difficulty providing care

    d. When there is danger such as from fire, poisonous fumes, or an unstable structure

2. Which of the following information should you obtain in your interview of this victim while obtaining a SAMPLE history?

    a. Allergies, current medications, pertinent past history

    b. Name, age, religion

    c. Age, address, where his parents are

    d. What happened, medical conditions, vital signs

3. When performing the physical exam, what four items will you check when using the mnemonic DOTS during the physical exam?

◆ SELF-ASSESSMENT

Circle the letter of the best answer.

1. Which one of the following victims should receive some form of care before you perform a physical exam?

   a. A conscious, cooperative victim

   b. A victim with a bruise on the head

   c. A victim bleeding severely from the neck

   d. A victim complaining of pain in an ankle

2. Which of the following techniques would you use in performing a physical examination of an adult victim?

   a. Visually inspect the entire body, starting with the head.

   b. Gently run your hands over each arm and leg to feel for possible broken bones.

   c. Ask the victim to take a deep breath and exhale, unless he or she complains of chest pain.

   d. All of the above.

3. The purpose of the physical exam is to—

   a. Find injuries or conditions that are not immediately life threatening.

   b. Determine if the victim is bleeding severely.

   c. Size up the scene for hazardous conditions.

   d. Find out the victim's name and address.

4. Why should you do an initial assessment in every emergency situation?

   a. Because it will protect you from legal liability

   b. Because it identifies conditions that are an immediate threat to life

   c. Because it will enable you to protect the victim and bystanders from dangers at the scene

   d. All of the above

5. Which of the following is an example of an immediately life-threatening problem?

   a. A 22-year-old man who, since last night, has had a fever and has vomited three times

   b. A 70-year-old jogger experiencing severe knee pain after her morning run

   c. A 40-year-old executive complaining that he has been experiencing a sharp pain in his side when he breathes in deeply

   d. A 6-year-old girl who was pulled unconscious from a swimming pool

6. In sizing up the scene of an emergency, you must consider four components. Three of these are scene safety, mechanism of injury/nature of illness, and the number of victims. What is the fourth component?

   a. The location of any vehicles blocking the path of arriving EMS personnel

   b. Whether there is fire or smoke present

   c. The time of the emergency

   d. The resources needed

7. The normal breathing rate for an adult is between _____ and _____ breaths per minute.

   a. 5,10

   b. 6,12

   c. 12,20

   d. 20,24

8. When should you perform a physical exam?

   a. When caring for a conscious, cooperative victim

   b. When caring for a victim who has an obvious head injury

   c. When caring for a victim who is unresponsive and vomiting

   d. a and b

9. The signs and symptoms of abnormal breathing include—

   a. Gasping for air.

   b. Quiet, regular breaths.

   c. Whistling, crowing, or gurgling sounds.

   d. a and c.

10. You are walking with a neighbor when he steps off a curb and turns his ankle. He appears to have injured the ankle but does not want you to call for help. After a few minutes he wants to stand up. What should you do?

    a. Call EMS personnel; he may have a broken ankle.

    b. Get your car and drive him to the hospital.

    c. Help him stand up and reassess his condition.

    d. Call his doctor for advice.

Notes

PRACTICE SESSION: *Performing an Initial Assessment*

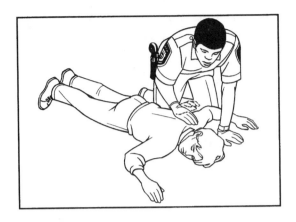

☐ **Check level of consciousness**
- ◆ Tap and gently shake person.
- ◆ Shout, "Are you OK?"

If victim does not respond...

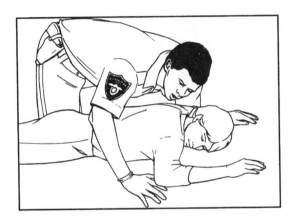

☐ **Check for breathing**
- ◆ Look, listen, and feel for about 5 seconds.

If not breathing or you cannot tell...

- ◆ Position victim onto back while supporting the head and back.

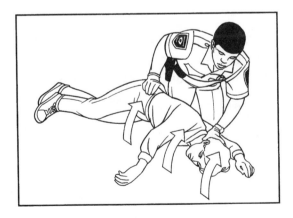

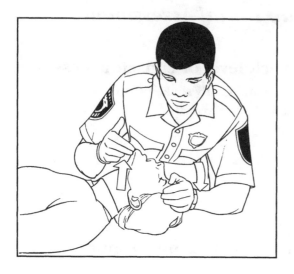

- Open the airway.
- Tilt head back and lift chin for victims without trauma; for trauma victims, use jaw thrust without head lift.

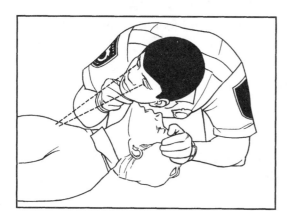

- Recheck breathing.
- Look, listen, and feel for about 5 seconds.

If person is not breathing...

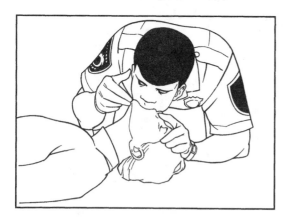

- Keep head tilted back.
- Pinch nose shut.
- Seal your lips tightly around person's mouth.
- Give 2 slow full breaths, each lasting about 2 seconds. Use a barrier device whenever available.

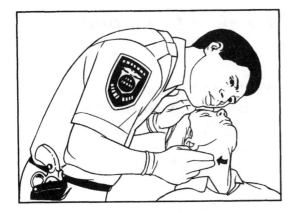

☐ Check for pulse

- ◆ Locate Adam's apple.
- ◆ Slide fingers down into groove of neck on side close to you.
- ◆ Feel for pulse.

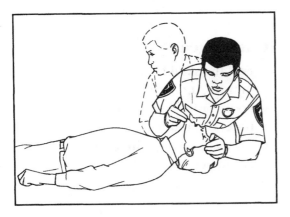

☐ Check for severe bleeding and skin characteristics

- ◆ Look from head to toe for severe bleeding.
- ◆ If the person has a pulse and is breathing, look at and feel the victim's skin to determine color, temperature and moisture.

If victim has a pulse and is not breathing...

- ◆ **Do rescue breathing.**

If victim does not have a pulse...

- ◆ **Begin CPR.**

If victim has a pulse and is breathing...

- ◆ **Perform a physical exam and SAMPLE history if able to do so.**

PRACTICE SESSION: *Performing a Physical Exam and SAMPLE History*

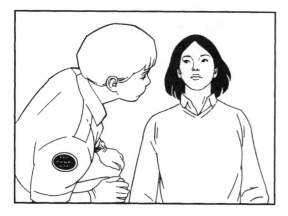

☐ **Perform a physical exam beginning with the head**

- ◆ As you conduct the physical exam, look and feel for—
  - Deformity.
  - Open injuries.
  - Tenderness.
  - Swelling.

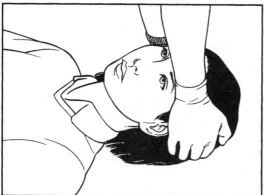

☐ **Check head**

- ◆ Feel the skull for deformities, open injuries, tenderness and swelling.
- ◆ Look for fluid or blood in the ears, nose, or mouth.
- ◆ Note any changes in level of consciousness.

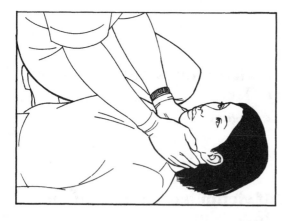

☐ **Check neck**

- ◆ Feel sides and back of the neck.
- ◆ If no discomfort and no suspected injury to the neck, ask person to move head slowly from side to side.

Check shoulders

- Feel shoulders and collarbone.
- Ask person to shrug shoulders.

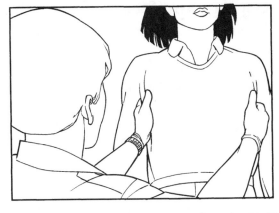

Check chest

- Feel ribs and sternum.
- Ask person to take deep breath and blow air out.
- Listen for signs of difficulty breathing.

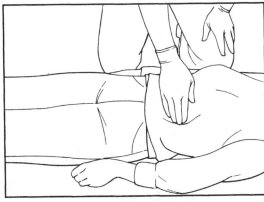

Check abdomen

- Apply slight pressure to each side of the abdomen, high and low.

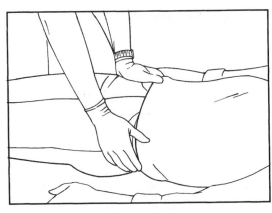

Check pelvis

- Push down and in on both sides of the pelvis with your hands.

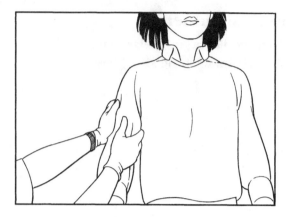

☐ **Check arms and hands**

- ◆ Feel both sides of each arm and hand, one at a time.
- ◆ Ask person to try to move fingers, hands, and arms.

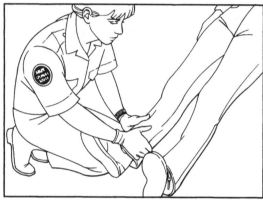

☐ **Check legs and feet**

- ◆ Feel both sides of each leg and foot, one at a time.
- ◆ Ask person to try to—
  - • Move toes, foot, ankle.
  - • Bend leg.

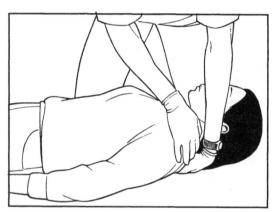

☐ **Check back**

- ◆ Gently reach under person and feel the back.

☐ **Obtain SAMPLE history**

- ◆ Interview the victim to obtain SAMPLE history.
- ◆ Ask—
  - • For any signs and symptoms.
  - • If he or she has any allergies.
  - • If he or she is taking any medications.
  - • If he or she has any previous medical conditions.
  - • When was the last time he or she ate.
  - • What he or she was doing before and at the time of the injury or illness.

Perform an on-going assessment until more advanced medical personnel arrive...

If there are no signs or symptoms of injury or illness and the person can move body parts without pain or discomfort...

- ◆ Keep watching the person's LOC, breathing, pulse, and skin characteristics.
- ◆ If any life-threatening problems develop, stop whatever you are doing and provide care immediately.

If person is unable to move a body part, is experiencing pain on movement, or level of consciousness is not normal...

- ◆ Recheck breathing and pulse.
- ◆ Help person rest in most comfortable position.
- ◆ Prevent person from becoming chilled or over heated.
- ◆ Reassure person.

PRACTICE SESSION: *Blood Pressure Measurement (Palpation)*

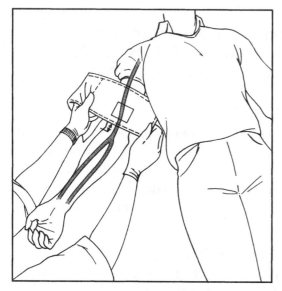

☐ **Position cuff**

- ◆ Place cuff 1 inch above crease in elbow.
- ◆ Center cuff over brachial artery.

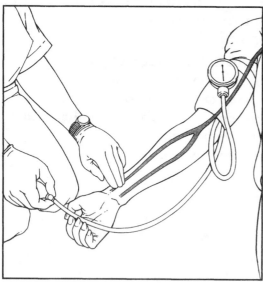

☐ **Locate radial pulse**

- ◆ Feel for pulse on thumb side of wrist.

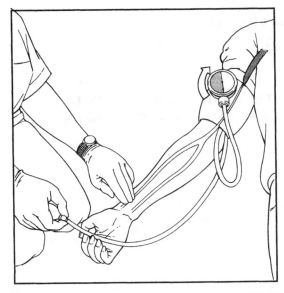

☐ Inflate cuff beyond point where pulse disappears

- ◆ Inflate 20 mm Hg beyond point where pulse disappears.

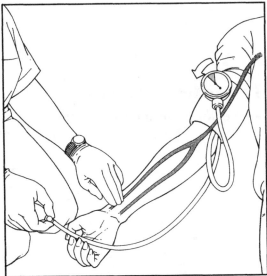

☐ Deflate cuff until pulse returns

- ◆ Deflate slowly—2 mm Hg/sec until pulse returns.
- ◆ Note point at which pulse returns.
- ◆ Quickly deflate cuff completely by opening the valve.

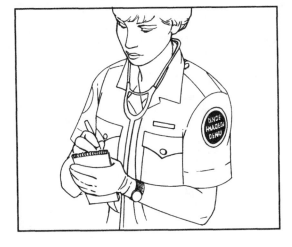

☐ Record approximate systolic pressure

PRACTICE SESSION: *Blood Pressure Measurement (Auscultation)*

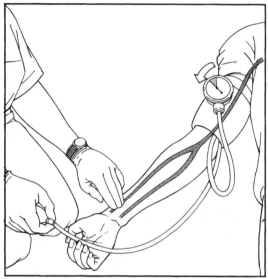

☐ **Determine approximate systolic blood pressure**

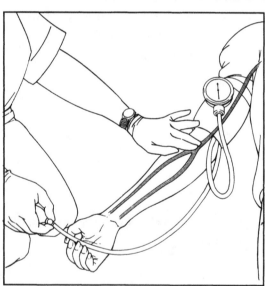

☐ **Locate brachial pulse**
- ◆ Feel for pulse at crease in elbow.

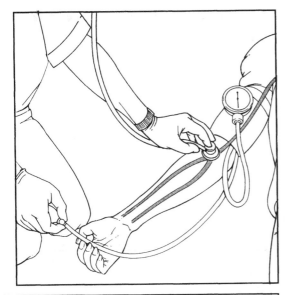

☐ Position stethoscope

- ◆ Place diaphragm over brachial pulse.

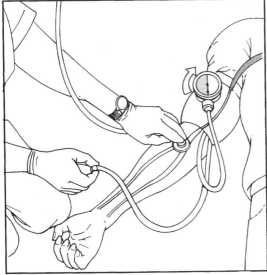

☐ Inflate cuff beyond approximate systolic pressure

- ◆ Inflate 20 mm Hg beyond approximate systolic pressure.

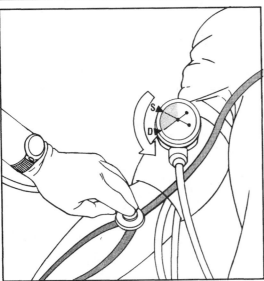

☐ Deflate cuff until pulse is heard

- ◆ Deflate slowly — 2 mm Hg/sec. Note point at which pulse is first heard (systolic pressure).

☐ Continue deflating cuff until pulse is no longer heard

- ◆ Note point at which pulse disappears (diastolic pressure).
- ◆ Quickly deflate cuff.

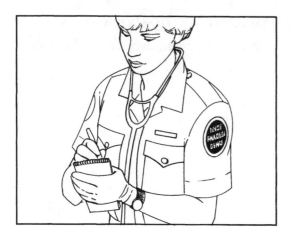

☐ **Record systolic and diastolic pressures**

Notes

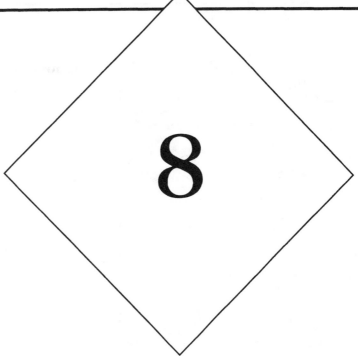

Breathing
Emergencies

◆ SUMMARY

In Chapter 8, you learned how to recognize and provide care for breathing emergencies. You now know to look for a breathing emergency in the initial assessment because such an emergency can be life threatening. You learned the signs and symptoms of respiratory distress and respiratory arrest, and the appropriate care for each condition. You also learned the basic techniques for rescue breathing and for special situations. Finally, you learned how to care for choking victims, both conscious and unconscious. By knowing how to care for breathing emergencies, you are better prepared to care for other emergencies.

◆ OUTLINE

◆ LEARNING ACTIVITIES

Matching

Match each term with its definition. Write its letter on the line in front of the definition.

Terms

a. Respiratory distress

b. Airway obstruction

c. Respiratory arrest

d. Aspiration

e. Head-tilt/chin-lift

f. Rescue breathing

Definitions

1. _____ A technique for opening the airway

2. _____ A condition in which breathing has stopped

3. _____ A blockage that prevents air from reaching the lungs

4. _____ A condition in which breathing is difficult

5. _____ Taking blood, saliva, vomit, or other foreign matter into the lungs

6. _____ Technique of breathing air into a victim's lungs, supplying him or her with adequate oxygen

True/False

Circle T if the statement is true; circle F if it is false.

1. T F When giving care to a conscious choking child, you give 5 abdominal thrusts followed by 5 back blows.

2. T F You should check the victim for a pulse once every minute while providing rescue breathing.

3. T F Drinking alcohol with meals helps people relax and reduces the risk of choking.

4. T F An individual in respiratory distress may sometimes breathe more slowly than normal.

5. T F If a victim of asthma has his or her prescribed medication available, you should assist the victim in taking it, if you are authorized to do so.

6. T F When performing rescue breathing, you should push down on the forehead and lift up on the chin to keep the airway open.

7. T F By leaning forward and pressing the abdomen over a chairback, railing, or kitchen counter, a choking victim can give himself or herself abdominal thrusts.

8. T F Ringing in the ears is one sign of respiratory distress.

9. T F You should always perform a finger sweep in the mouth of an unconscious choking infant.

10. T F You should provide rescue breathing to a conscious victim with an obstructed airway.

11. T F If the 2 slow breaths you deliver to an unconscious choking victim do not go in, you should retilt the head and deliver 2 slow breaths again.

12. T F Seeing the victim's chest rise and fall is a good indicator that your breaths are entering the victim's lungs during rescue breathing.

13. T F For you to give abdominal thrusts to a conscious adult choking victim, he or she must be standing.

14. T F To care for a conscious choking infant, deliver 5 back blows followed by 5 chest thrusts.

15. T F A victim who has a pulse does not require rescue breathing.

Short Answer

Read each statement or question and write the correct answer or answers in the space provided.

1. List five situations in which it is appropriate for you to stop rescue breathing.

2. List five common causes of choking.

3. List at least six signs and symptoms of respiratory distress.

4. Number each step pictured in the order in which it is performed. Write the step shown in each picture next to its number.

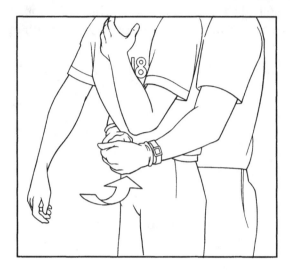

a. _____ _____

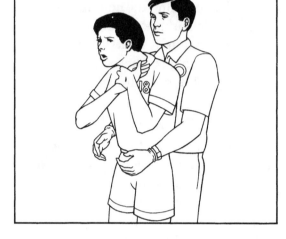

b. _____ _____

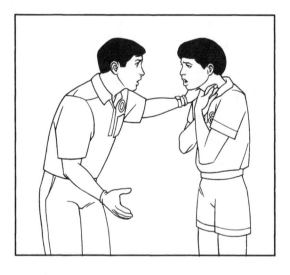

c. _____ _____

d. _____ _____

5. Number each step pictured in the order
    in which it is performed. Write the
    step shown in each picture next to its
    number.

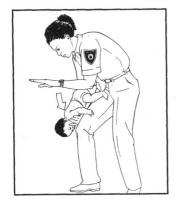

a. _____ _____

_____

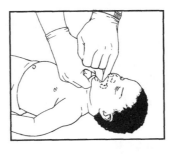

b. _____ _____

_____

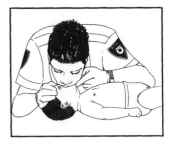

c. _____ _____

_____

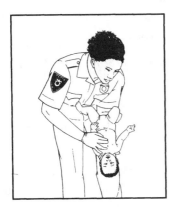

d. _____ _____

_____

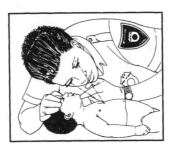

e. _____ _____

_____

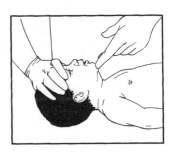

f. _____ _____

_____

◆ CASE STUDIES

Read the case studies and answer the questions that follow.

Case 8.1

You are summoned to a home where you find a 3-month-old baby girl in her crib, struggling and cyanotic. You hear very high-pitched wheezes but do not see any rise and fall of the chest or hear or feel any air going in and out at the mouth and nose. She is not crying.

1. If you suspect an obstructed airway, what will you do first to try to clear the obstruction from the airway?

   a. Give two slow breaths.

   b. Tilt her head back and pull up on the jaw.

   c. Administer 5 chest thrusts using two fingers.

   d. Give 5 back blows.

2. Describe how you will position the infant to begin your emergency care.

3. T   F   When you deliver back blows or chest thrusts to this infant, her head should be kept higher than the rest of her body.

4. How would you find the correct hand position for delivering chest thrusts to this infant?

5. T   F   When you deliver rescue breathing to this infant, you should cover her nose and mouth with your mouth to give the breaths.

Case 8.2

At a scene where a car crashed into a utility pole, you find the driver unconscious on the ground. He is bleeding slightly from wounds on his forehead and left cheek and does not appear to be breathing.

1. How should you first attempt to open his airway?

   a. Use the head-tilt/chin-lift to move his tongue away from the back of the throat.

   b. Pull his lower jaw forward by putting your thumb in his mouth and your fingers on the jaw.

   c. Lift his chin using a two-handed jaw-thrust maneuver without tilting the head back.

   d. Turn his head to the side and clear any blood and foreign matter from his mouth.

2. The preferred method of rescue breathing to use with this victim is—

    a. Mouth-to-mouth.

    b. Mouth-to-mouth and nose.

    c. Mouth-to-nose.

    d. Mouth-to-mask.

3. Describe what you would do if the victim vomited during your attempts at rescue breathing.

4. T F You should breathe with quick, forceful breaths to make the victim's chest rise and clear the airway.

5. As you continue rescue breathing, how often would you recheck the pulse?

6. If this victim were a child instead of an adult, how often would you provide rescue breathing?

    a. Once every second

    b. Once every 3 seconds

    c. Once every 5 seconds

    d. Once every minute

◆ **SELF-ASSESSMENT**

Circle the letter of the best answer.

1. When giving back blows to a choking infant, the head should be—

    a. Higher than the chest.

    b. Turned to the side.

    c. Lower than the chest.

    d. Resting on your thigh.

2. When performing rescue breathing, what should you do after giving the first 2 slow breaths?

    a. Reposition the head.

    b. Check for a pulse.

    c. Check for consciousness.

    d. Repeat the two breaths.

3. If the victim's airway is not adequately opened and breaths are delivered forcefully during rescue breathing, what will happen?

    a. Air will go into the victim's stomach.

    b. Gastric distention can cause vomiting.

    c. Adequate oxygen may not reach into the victim's lungs.

    d. All of the above.

4. What should you do when a victim is breathing rapidly and you are certain it is caused by emotion?

    a. Place the victim on one side to ease breathing.

    b. Administer oxygen if it is available and you are trained to do so.

    c. Ask the victim to try to breathe as slow as you are breathing.

    d. Assist the victim in taking his or her prescribed medication if you are authorized to do so.

5. When you provide rescue breathing to a victim, you are—

   a. Artificially circulating oxygenated blood to the body cells.

   b. Supplementing the air the victim is already breathing.

   c. Supplying the victim with oxygen necessary for survival.

   d. All of the above.

6. Signs of respiratory distress include—

   a. Noisy breathing.

   b. Rapid or slow breathing.

   c. Constricted pupils.

   d. a and b.

7. Which is a common cause of choking?

   a. Drinking alcohol before or during meals

   b. Wearing dentures

   c. Eating small pieces of well-chewed food

   d. a and b

8. After discovering that your first 2 breaths are not causing the victim's chest to rise, what should you do?

   a. Retilt the head and give breaths again.

   b. Begin rescue breathing.

   c. Give 2 more breaths with greater force.

   d. Do a finger sweep.

9. Which would be included in your care for an unconscious choking child?

   a. Positioning the child on his or her back

   b. Repeated abdominal thrusts until the object is dislodged

   c. Doing a finger sweep if you see the object

   d. a and c

10. Which technique is used to provide oxygen to a victim of respiratory arrest?

    a. Mechanical breathing

    b. Oxygen supplementation by mask

    c. Rescue breathing

    d. Abdominal thrusts

Notes

Notes

PRACTICE SESSION: *Rescue Breathing for an Adult or Child*

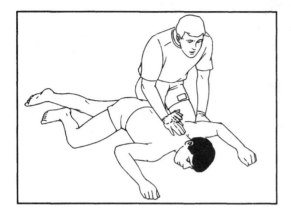

☐ **Check for consciousness**

- ◆ Tap and gently shake person.
- ◆ Shout, "Are you OK?"

If person does not respond...

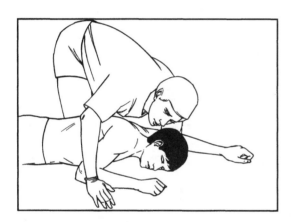

☐ **Check for breathing**

- ◆ Look, listen, and feel for about 5 seconds.

If not breathing or you cannot tell...

- ◆ Roll person onto back while supporting the head and back.

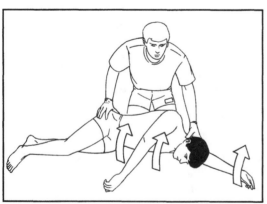

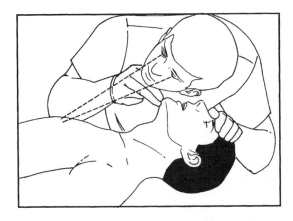

- ◆ Open the airway.
- ◆ Tilt head back and lift chin.
- ◆ Recheck breathing.
- ◆ Look, listen, and feel for about 5 seconds.

If person is not breathing...

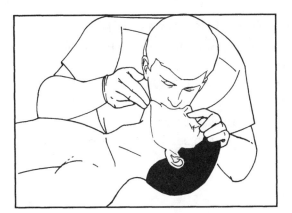

- ◆ Keep head tilted back.
- ◆ Pinch nose shut.
- ◆ Seal your lips tightly around person's mouth.
- ◆ Give 2 slow breaths, each lasting about 1 1/2 seconds. Use a barrier device whenever possible.
- ◆ Watch to see that the breaths go in.

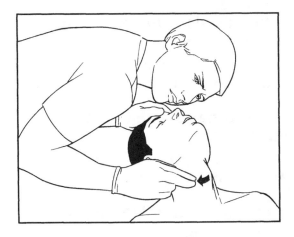

☐ Check for pulse

- ◆ Locate Adam's apple.
- ◆ Slide fingers down into groove of neck on side closer to you.
- ◆ Feel for carotid pulse for 5 to 10 seconds.

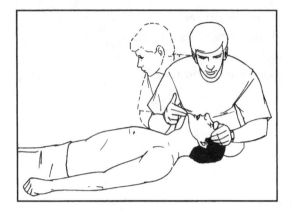

☐ Check for severe bleeding

- ◆ Look from head to toe for severe bleeding.

If person has a pulse and is not breathing...

- ◆ Do rescue breathing.

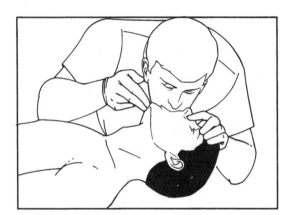

☐ Begin rescue breathing

- ◆ Maintain open airway with head-tilt/chin-lift.
- ◆ Pinch nose shut.
- ◆ Give 1 slow breath every 5 seconds. (1 slow breath every 3 seconds for a child).
- ◆ Watch chest to see that your breaths go in.

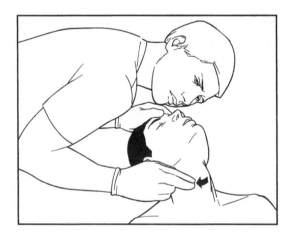

☐ Recheck pulse and breathing every minute

- ◆ Feel for pulse for about 5 seconds.
- ◆ Look, listen, and feel for breathing.

If person has a pulse and is breathing...

- ◆ Keep airway open.
- ◆ Monitor breathing.

If person has a pulse but is still not breathing...

- ◆ Continue rescue breathing.

If person does not have a pulse and is not breathing...

- ◆ Begin CPR.

PRACTICE SESSION: *Rescue Breathing for an Infant*

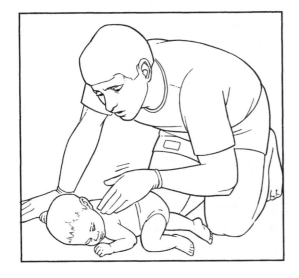

☐ **Check for consciousness**

- ◆ Tap and gently shake infant's shoulder.

If infant does not respond...

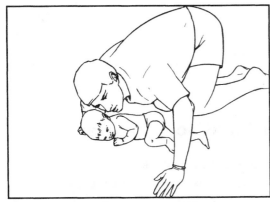

☐ **Check for breathing**

- ◆ Look, listen, and feel for about 5 seconds.

If not breathing or you cannot tell...

- ◆ Position infant onto back while supporting the head and back.

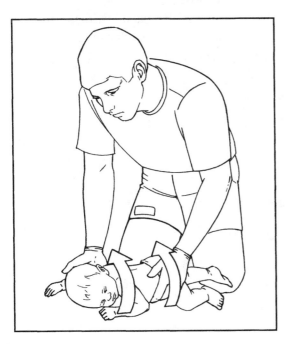

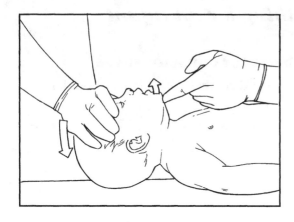

- ◆ Open the airway.
- ◆ Tilt head back and lift chin.

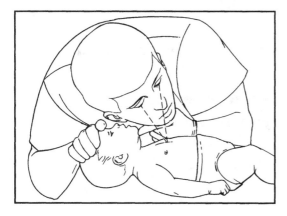

- ◆ Recheck breathing.
- ◆ Look, listen, and feel for about 5 seconds.

If infant is not breathing ...

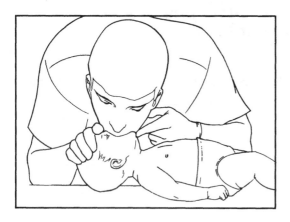

- ◆ Keep head tilted back.
- ◆ Seal your lips tightly around infant's mouth and nose.
- ◆ Give 2 slow breaths, each lasting about 1 1/2 seconds. Use a barrier device whenever possible.
- ◆ Watch to see that the breaths go in.

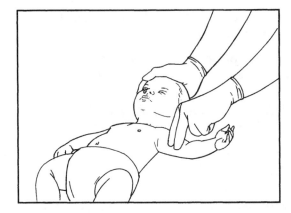

☐ **Check for pulse**

- ◆ Locate brachial pulse.
- ◆ Place fingers on the inside of upper arm midway between elbow and shoulder.
- ◆ Feel for pulse for 5 to 10 seconds.

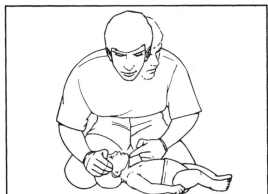

☐ **Check for severe bleeding**

- ◆ Look from head to toe for severe bleeding.

If infant has a pulse and is not breathing...

- ◆ Do rescue breathing.

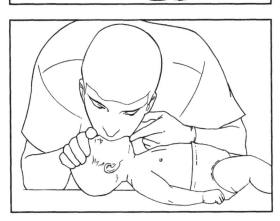

☐ **Begin rescue breathing**

- ◆ Maintain open airway with head-tilt/chin-lift.
- ◆ Give 1 slow breath every 3 seconds.
- ◆ Watch chest to see that your breaths go in.
- ◆ Continue for 1 minute—about 20 breaths.

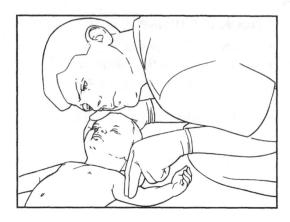

☐ **Recheck pulse and breathing every minute**

- ◆ Feel for pulse for about 5 seconds.
- ◆ Look, listen, and feel for breathing.

If infant has a pulse and is breathing...

- ◆ **Keep airway open.**
- ◆ **Monitor breathing.**

If infant has a pulse but is still not breathing...

- ◆ **Continue rescue breathing.**

If infant does not have a pulse and is not breathing...

- ◆ **Begin CPR.**

PRACTICE SESSION: ***Care for an Unconscious Adult or Child with a Complete Airway Obstruction***

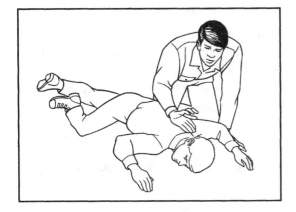

☐ Check for consciousness

- ◆ Tap and gently shake person.
- ◆ Shout, "Are you OK?"

If person does not respond...

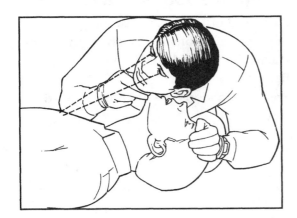

☐ Check for breathing

- ◆ Look, listen, and feel for about 5 seconds.

If not breathing or you cannot tell...

- ◆ Roll person as a single unit, while supporting the head and neck.
- ◆ Open the airway.
- ◆ Tilt head back and lift chin.
- ◆ Recheck breathing.
- ◆ Look, listen, and feel for about 5 seconds.

If person is not breathing...

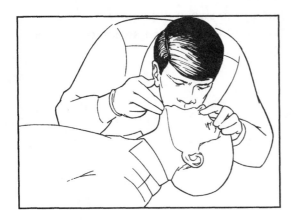

- ◆ Keep head tilted back.
- ◆ Pinch nose shut.
- ◆ Seal your lips tightly around person's mouth.
- ◆ Give 2 slow breaths, each lasting about 1 1/2 seconds. Use a barrier device whenever possible.
- ◆ Watch to see that the breaths go in.

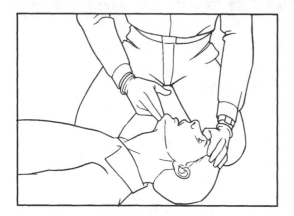

If breaths do not go in...

☐ **Retilt person's head and try 2 slow breaths again**

- ◆ Tilt head farther back.
- ◆ Pinch nose shut and seal your lips tightly around person's mouth.
- ◆ Reattempt 2 slow breaths, each lasting about 1 1/2 seconds.

If breaths still do not go in...

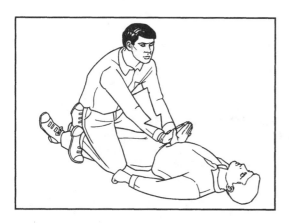

☐ **Give up to 5 abdominal thrusts**

- ◆ Place heel of 1 hand against middle of person's abdomen, just above the navel.
- ◆ Place other hand directly on top of first hand.
- ◆ Press into abdomen with quick upward thrusts.

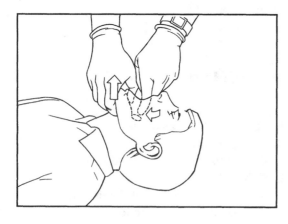

☐ **Do finger sweep** (simulate)

- ◆ Grasp both tongue and lower jaw between your thumb and fingers and lift jaw.
- ◆ Slide finger down inside of cheek to base of tongue.
- ◆ Attempt to sweep object out.
- ◆ For a child, do a finger sweep only if you see the object.

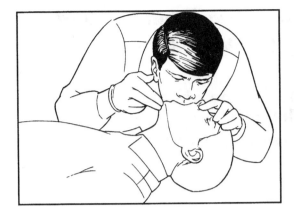

☐ Open airway and give 2 slow breaths

- ◆ Tilt head back.
- ◆ Pinch nose shut.
- ◆ Seal your lips tightly around person's mouth.
- ◆ Breaths should last about 1 1/2 seconds.
- ◆ Watch chest to see if your breaths go in.

If breaths still do not go in...

- ◆ **Retilt the head and reattempt breaths.**
- ◆ **Continue with sequence of thrusts, finger sweeps, head tilt, 2 slow breaths, head retilt, and 2 slow breaths until...**
  - • **Obstruction is removed.**
  - • **Person starts to breathe or cough.**
  - • **More advanced medical personnel arrive and take over.**

If breaths go in...

- ◆ **Check pulse and breathing.**
- ◆ **If person has pulse, but is not breathing, do rescue breathing.**
- ◆ **If person does not have pulse and is not breathing, do CPR.**
- ◆ **Check for and control severe bleeding.**

PRACTICE SESSION: *Care for a Conscious Adult or Child with an Airway Obstruction*

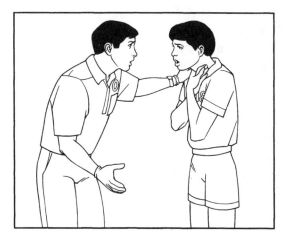

☐ **Determine whether person is choking**

♦ Ask, "Are you choking?"

If person is choking...

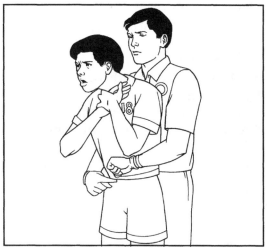

☐ **Give abdominal thrusts**

♦ Position yourself to give abdominal thrusts.
♦ Wrap your arms around person's waist.
♦ With one hand find the navel. With the other hand make a fist.
♦ Place thumb side of fist against middle of person's abdomen just above the navel and well below lower tip of breastbone.
♦ Grasp fist with your other hand.

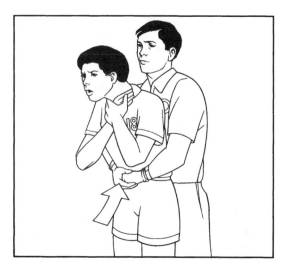

♦ Press fist into person's abdomen with a quick upward thrust.
♦ Each thrust should be a separate and distinct attempt to dislodge the object.

Repeat abdominal thrusts until...

♦ **Object is expelled.**
♦ **Person starts to breathe or cough forcefully.**
♦ **Person becomes unconscious.**
♦ **More advanced medical personnel arrive and take over.**

PRACTICE SESSION: *Care for an Unconscious Infant with a Complete Airway Obstruction*

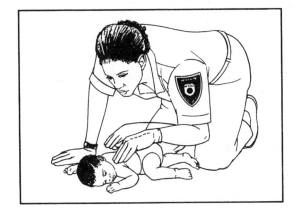

☐ **Check for consciousness**

- ◆ Tap and gently shake infant's shoulder.

If infant does not respond...

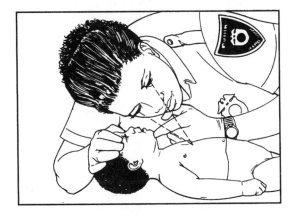

☐ **Check for breathing**

- ◆ Look, listen, and feel for about 5 seconds.

If not breathing or you cannot tell...

- ◆ Roll infant on back while supporting the head and neck.
- ◆ Open the airway.
- ◆ Tilt head back and lift chin.
- ◆ Recheck breathing.
- ◆ Look, listen, and feel for about 5 seconds.

If infant is not breathing...

- ◆ Keep head tilted back.
- ◆ Seal your lips tightly around infant's mouth and nose.
- ◆ Give 2 slow breaths, each lasting about 1 1/2 seconds.
- ◆ Watch to see that the breaths go in.

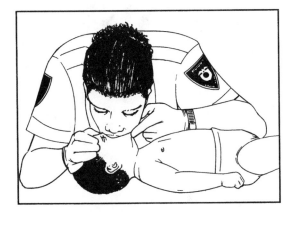

If breaths do not go in...

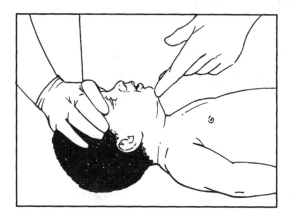

☐ **Retilt infant's head and try 2 slow breaths again.**

- ◆ Tilt infant's head farther back.
- ◆ Seal your lips tightly around infant's mouth and nose.
- ◆ Give 2 slow breaths, each lasting about 1 1/2 seconds.

If breaths still do not go in...

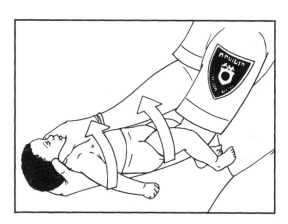

☐ **Give 5 back blows**

- ◆ Position infant facedown on forearm.
- ◆ Lower forearm onto thigh.
- ◆ Infant's head should be lower than feet.

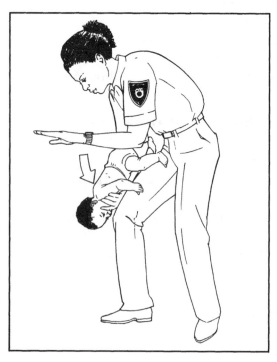

- ◆ Using the heel of your hand, give forceful back blows between infant's shoulder blades, 5 times.
- ◆ Each blow should be a separate and distinct attempt to dislodge the object.

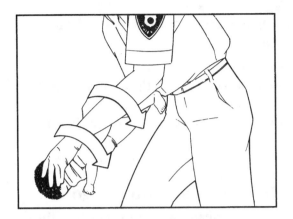

☐ **Give 5 chest thrusts**

- ◆ Position infant faceup on forearm.
- ◆ Lower forearm onto thigh.

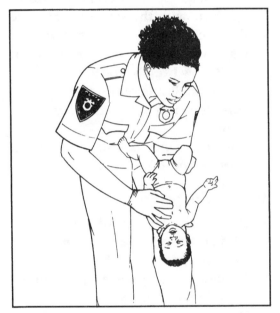

- ◆ Locate position for chest thrusts.
- ◆ Using pads of two fingers, smoothly compress breastbone 1/2 to 1 inch, 5 times.
- ◆ Each thrust should be a separate and distinct attempt to dislodge the object.

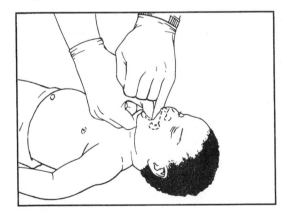

☐ **Do foreign-body check**

- ◆ Grasp both tongue and lower jaw between your thumb and fingers and lift jaw.
- ◆ If object can be seen, slide little finger down inside of cheek to base of tongue.
- ◆ Attempt to sweep object out.

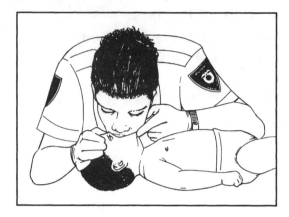

☐ **Open airway and give 2 slow breaths**

- ◆ Tilt head back.
- ◆ Seal your lips tightly around infant's mouth and nose.
- ◆ Give 2 slow breaths, each lasting about 1 1/2 seconds.
- ◆ Watch to see if your breaths go in.

If breaths still do not go in...

- ◆ **Retilt head and reattempt breaths. Continue with the sequence of back blows, chest thrusts, finger sweeps, head tilt, 2 slow breaths, head retilt, and 2 slow breaths until...**
  - • **Obstruction is removed.**
  - • **Infant starts to breathe, cry, or cough.**
  - • **More advanced medical personnel arrive and take over.**

If breaths go in...

- ◆ **Check pulse and breathing.**
- ◆ **If infant has a pulse, but is not breathing, do rescue breathing.**
- ◆ **If infant does not have a pulse and is not breathing, do CPR.**
- ◆ **Check and control severe bleeding.**

Notes

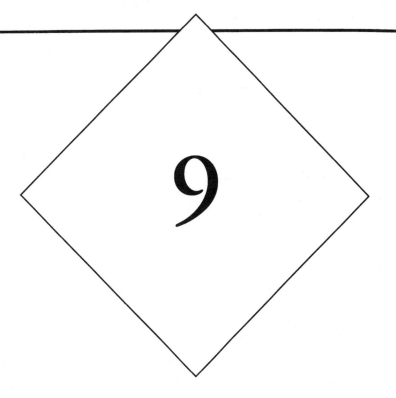

Breathing Devices

◆ SUMMARY

Breathing devices can make the emergency care you provide safer, easier, and more effective. Suction equipment helps clear the airway of substances, such as water, blood, saliva, or vomit. Oral and nasal airways help maintain an open airway by keeping the tongue away from the back of the throat. The use of supplemental oxygen can relieve pain and breathing discomfort. Barrier shields, resuscitation masks, and BVMs are the most appropriate devices for first responders to use when ventilating a victim. They can significantly increase the oxygen concentration that an ill or injured person needs, help ventilate a nonbreathing person, and reduce the likelihood of disease transmission.

Breathing devices, such as the ones discussed in this chapter, are appropriate for almost all types of injury or illness in which breathing may be impaired. Knowing how to use these devices will enable you to provide more effective care until more advanced medical personnel arrive.

◆ OUTLINE

Any items marked with ** indicate information found only in the Enrichment section of the text.

◆ LEARNING ACTIVITIES

Matching

Match each term with its definition. Write its letter on the line in front of the definition.

Terms

a. Resuscitation mask

b. Suctioning

c. Bag-valve-mask (BVM) resuscitator

d. Oral airway

e. Nasal airway

Definitions

1. _____ The process of removing matter from a victim's mouth or throat by means of a mechanical or manual device

2. _____ A ventilation device best used by two rescuers because one person may have difficulty keeping the airway open while still maintaining a tight enough seal

3. _____ A device inserted into the mouth of an unconscious victim to keep the tongue from obstructing the airway

4. _____ A pliable, dome-shaped device that fits over the victim's nose and mouth used for rescue breathing

5. _____ A device inserted into the nose of a conscious or unconscious victim to help maintain an open airway

**Matching

Match each term with its definition. Write its letter on the line in front of the definition.

Terms

a. Flowmeter

b. Nasal cannula

c. Oxygen cylinder

d. Nonrebreather mask

e. Pressure regulator

Definitions

1. _____ A device that regulates oxygen delivery in liters per minute (lpm)

2. _____ A device that administers oxygen to a victim who is breathing, but can be ineffective in a victim who has a bad cold

3. _____ A piece of equipment with an internal pressure of approximately 2000 pounds per square inch

4. _____ A device attached to an oxygen cylinder that reduces the delivery pressure to a safe level

5. _____ A type of oxygen mask capable of delivering a high concentration of oxygen to a breathing victim

True/False

Circle T if the statement is true; circle F if it is false.

1. T F For a proper seal, one rim of the resuscitation mask should be placed between the victim's lower lip and chin.

2. T F Gagging is a normal response from a victim in whom you are inserting an oropharyngeal airway and should not interrupt the process.

3. T F One of the advantages of breathing devices is that they allow the rescuer to deliver a higher concentration of oxygen to the victim than simple rescue breathing.

4. T F The main purpose of an oral airway is to keep the victim's tongue from blocking the airway.

5. T F It is easy for a single rescuer to maintain a tight seal on the victim's face when using a bag-valve-mask resuscitator.

6. T F A nasal airway can only be used in an unresponsive victim.

7. T F When using suction, you should insert the suction tip far back in the throat, beyond eyesight, to remove all matter.

8. T F Suctioning is used to clear foreign matter blocking the airway from the victim's mouth.

9. T F A resuscitation mask must be placed so that it covers the victim's mouth, but not the nose.

10. T F The mouth-to-mask method of resuscitation provides a barrier against disease transmission.

11. T F A resuscitation mask should not be used on a victim with facial injuries because of the potential for causing further damage.

12. T F If using a bag-valve-mask resuscitator alone, hold the mask in place by making a "C–clamp" with your index finger and thumb around the mask.

13. T F A victim should not be suctioned for more than 15 seconds at a time.

14. T F After you insert an oropharyngeal airway, place the flange end in the victim's mouth.

15. T F For a resuscitation mask to be effective, it should be made of a transparent pliable material.

16. T F A correctly sized nasal airway should extend from the tip of the nose to the earlobe.

**17. T F The oxygen cylinder should be turned on for 1 second after the O-ring has been put in place to remove any dirt or debris from the cylinder valve.

**18. T F The oxygen delivery device should be placed over the victim's face before oxygen begins to flow from the device.

19. T F A person who suffers a serious injury can benefit from supplemental oxygen.

20. T F Oxygen should not be administered around open flames or sparks.

Short Answer

Read each statement and write the correct answer or answers in the space provided.

1. What are the three steps to follow to maintain a good seal when using a resuscitation mask?

2. What are the six steps to follow when using a suction device?

** 3. The three items of equipment necessary for administration of supplemental oxygen are—

** 4. The four safety precautions you should follow when administering oxygen are—

** 5. The three unique characteristics that distinguish an oxygen cylinder from other gas storage cylinders are the—

◆ CASE STUDIES

Read the case studies and answer the questions that follow.

Case 9.1

You are summoned to a scene where you find a 20-year-old man unconscious on the floor. He has vomited, and much of the vomit remains in his mouth. He does not appear to be breathing.

1. **T F** The appropriate initial method for clearing the vomit from this man's mouth is to use a commercial suction device.

2. Describe how to measure the correct distance to insert a suction device to remove vomit from this victim's mouth.

3. After removing the vomit, you determine that the victim is not breathing. In providing artificial ventilation to this victim, how many ventilations per minute would you give?

   a. 6

   b. 12

   c. 24

   d. 36

** 4. Another first responder has arrived with oxygen and breathing devices. Which of the following breathing devices would allow you to supply this victim with the highest concentration of oxygen?

   a. Nasal cannula

   b. Resuscitation mask

   c. Nonrebreather mask

   d. Bag-valve-mask resuscitator

Case 9.2

You respond to a call for an unconscious victim. You are the first to arrive and find a woman lying on the floor, motionless. She is unconscious and not breathing, but does have a pulse.

1.   T F   Because of the possibility of disease transmission, you should use your available resuscitation mask to provide rescue breathing.

2.   T F   The proper placement for the resuscitation mask on this victim is to have one rim of the mask between her lower lip and chin and the opposite end of the mask covering her nose.

3. What concentration of oxygen can you deliver to this woman, using a flow of 10 or more liters per minute and using rescue breathing with a resuscitation mask?

   a. Approximately 16 percent

   b. Approximately 24 percent

   c. Approximately 35 percent

   d. Approximately 50 percent

◆ SELF-ASSESSMENT

Circle the letter of the best answer.

1. An oropharyngeal airway is the correct size if it extends from the victim's—

   a. Nose to the point of the chin.

   b. Nose tip to the earlobe.

   c. Earlobe to the corner of the mouth.

   d. Front teeth to the back of the tongue.

2. The first responder should assist a victim's breathing when the victim is—

   a. Breathing at a rate of more than 30 breaths per minute.

   b. Wheezing.

   c. Coughing with each breath.

   d. Conscious, but unable to respond to verbal questioning.

3. Which is an advantage of using a resuscitation mask to provide artificial ventilation?

   a. It reduces the volume of air needed to extend the victim's lungs.

   b. It prevents airway obstruction from occurring as a result of facial injuries.

   c. It reduces the risk of disease transmission between rescuer and victim.

   d. All of the above.

4. If you find that your hand is too small to completely compress the bag on a bag-valve-mask resuscitator, you can increase the amount of ventilation by—

   a. Compressing the bag against your thigh.

   b. Increasing the liter of flow oxygen to the bag.

   c. Pressing the mask more firmly to the victim's face.

   d. All of the above.

5. When using a resuscitation mask, the best way to maintain an open airway is to—

   a. Tilt the person's head back.

   b. Lift the jaw upward.

   c. Keep the person's mouth open.

   d. All of the above.

6. When you manually sweep secretions from a victim's mouth to clear the airway, you should—

   a. Lift the neck and tilt the head back.

   b. Use the triple airway maneuver.

   c. Roll the victim onto one side and sweep the mouth.

   d. Pull the jaw forward to move the tongue before sweeping the mouth.

7. Which step do you take when using a manual or mechanical suction device?

   a. Keep the victim's head turned to the side.

   b. Sweep debris from the mouth before suctioning.

   c. Suction for no more than 15 seconds at a time.

   d. All of the above.

** 8. A pressure regulator should not be lubricated with a petroleum product because of the danger of—

   a. Contamination of the oxygen.

   b. An explosion.

   c. Loosening the oxygen cylinder valve.

   d. Inaccurate readings from the oxygen flowmeter.

** 9. The O-ring should be placed on the oxygen cylinder—

   a. After the regulator is in place.

   b. After you have examined the pressure regulator.

   c. After you have opened the cylinder for 1 second.

   d. After you verified oxygen flow.

**10. Using a nasal cannula at a flow rate above 4 lpm for a prolonged period of time can cause —

   a. Nosebleed.

   b. Wheezing.

   c. Slow heart rate.

   d. All of the above.

Notes

PRACTICE SESSION: *Suctioning*

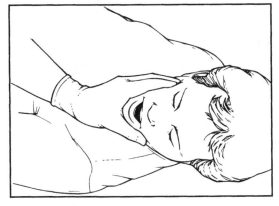

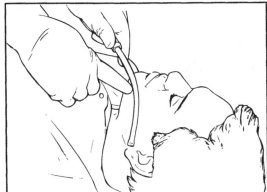

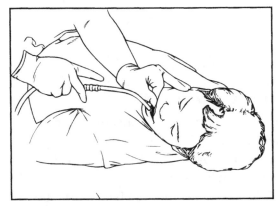

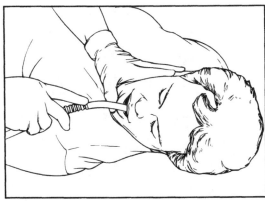

☐ **Position the person**

◆ Turn the person's head to one side
◆ If suspect head, neck, or back injury, roll the person onto one side while supporting the head and neck.
◆ Open the mouth

Sweep large debris from the mouth using your finger

☐ **Measure suction tip**

◆ Measure from the victim's earlobe to the corner of the mouth.
◆ Note the distance to prevent inserting suction tip too deeply.

Turn on machine and test it.

☐ **Suction the mouth**

◆ Insert suction tip into back of mouth.

◆ Apply suction as you withdraw the tip using a circular motion.
◆ Suction for no more than 15 seconds at a time.

PRACTICE SESSION: *Inserting an Oral Airway*

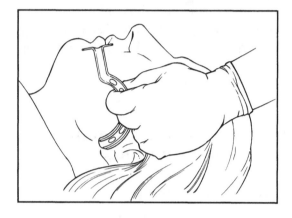

☐ **Select the proper size**

- ◆ Measure the airway from the victim's earlobe to the corner of the mouth.

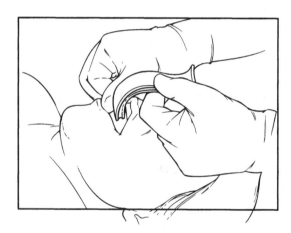

☐ **Open the victim's mouth**

- ◆ Use the cross finger technique to open the victim's mouth.

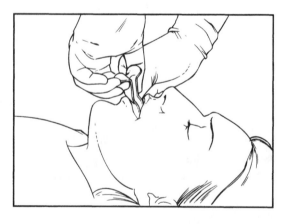

☐ **Insert the airway**

- ◆ Insert the airway with the curved end along the roof of the mouth.
- ◆ As tip approaches back of the mouth, rotate it a half turn.
- ◆ Slide the airway into the back of the throat.

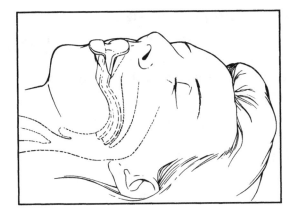

☐ Ensure correct placement

◆ The flange should rest on the victim's lips.
◆ If the victim begins to gag, immediately remove the airway.

PRACTICE SESSION: *Inserting a Nasal Airway*

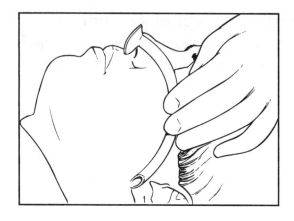

☐ ## Select the proper size
- ♦ Measure the nasal airway from the victim's earlobe to the tip of the nose.
- ♦ Ensure the diameter of the airway is not larger than the nostril.

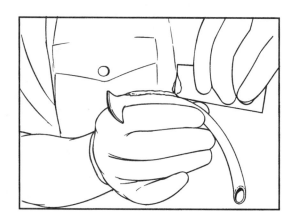

☐ ## Lubricate the airway
- ♦ Use a water-soluble lubricant to lubricate the airway prior to insertion.

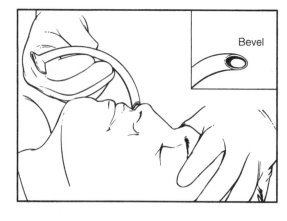

☐ ## Insert the airway
- ♦ Insert the airway into the nostril, with the bevel toward the septum.
- ♦ Advance the airway gently, straight in.
- ♦ If resistance is felt, do not force.

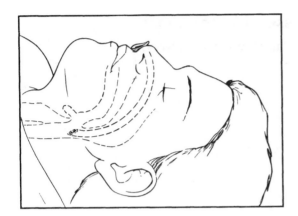

☐ **Ensure correct placement**

◆ The flange should rest on the nose.

PRACTICE SESSION: *Using a Resuscitation Mask for Rescue Breathing*

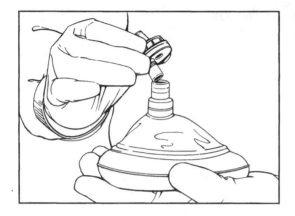

□ **Assemble the mask**
- ◆ Attach one-way valve to mask.

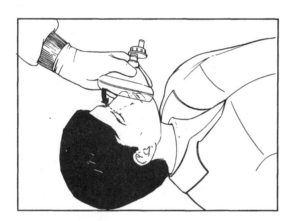

□ **Position the mask**
- ◆ Kneel behind victim's head.
- ◆ Place rim of mask between lower lip and chin.
- ◆ Cover victim's mouth and nose with mask.

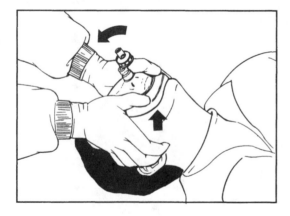

□ **Seal mask and open airway**
- ◆ Place your thumbs on each side of mask to hold it in place.
- ◆ Place fingers of both hands along victim's jawbone.
- ◆ Tilt head back.
- ◆ Apply downward pressure with thumbs while lifting the jaw upward with fingers.

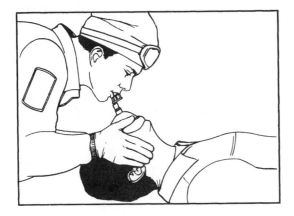

☐ **Begin rescue breathing**

◆ Give 1 slow breath about every 5 seconds (once about every 3 seconds for a child or infant).

◆ Watch chest to see that breaths go in.

◆ Recheck pulse every minute.

PRACTICE SESSION: *Using a Bag-Valve-Mask Resuscitator (BVM) for Rescue Breathing (Two Rescuers)*

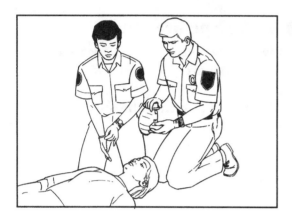

☐ **First rescuer—Assemble the BVM**
   ◆ Attach bag and valve to mask.

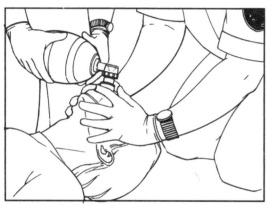

☐ **Position the mask**
   ◆ Place mask so that it covers victim's mouth and nose.

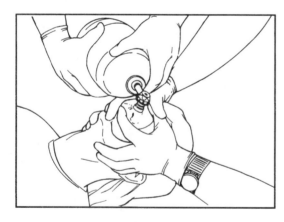

☐ **Seal mask and open airway**
   ◆ Place your thumbs on each side of mask to hold it in place.
   ◆ Place fingers of both hands along victim's jawbone.
   ◆ Tilt head back.
   ◆ Apply downward pressure with thumbs while lifting jaw upward with fingers.

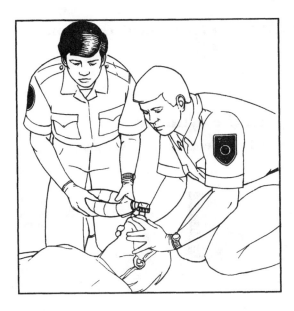

☐ Second rescuer—Begin ventilations

- ◆ Squeeze bag smoothly until victim's chest rises.
- ◆ Give 1 ventilation about every 5 seconds (once about every 3 seconds for a child or infant).
- ◆ Watch chest to see that ventilations go in.
- ◆ Recheck pulse every minute.

PRACTICE SESSION: *Oxygen Delivery* (Optional practice session)

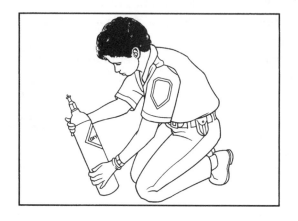

☐ **Check the cylinder**
   ◆ See that label is marked "Oxygen."

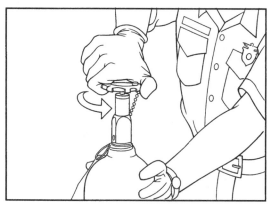

☐ **Clear the valve**
   ◆ Remove protective covering and save plastic gasket.
   ◆ Open cylinder for 1 second to clear the valve.

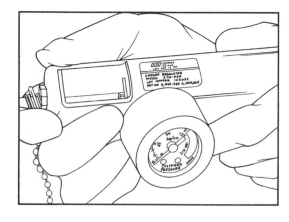

☐ **Attach the pressure regulator**
   ◆ See that it is marked "Oxygen Pressure Regulator."

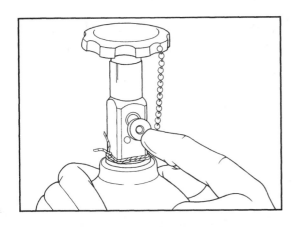

◆ Put plastic gasket into valve at top of cylinder.

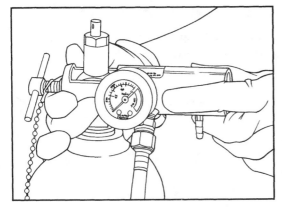

◆ Place regulator on cylinder.
◆ Seat the three metal prongs into valve.

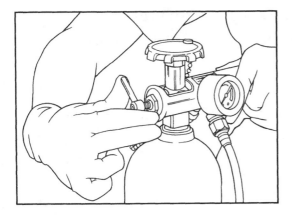

◆ Hand tighten screw until regulator is snug.

☐ **Open the cylinder 1 full turn**

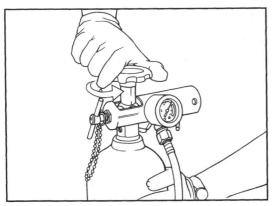

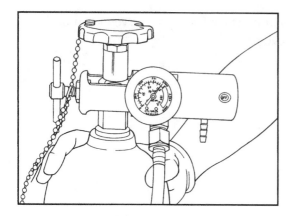

☐ **Check the pressure gauge**

- ◆ Determine how much pressure is in cylinder.

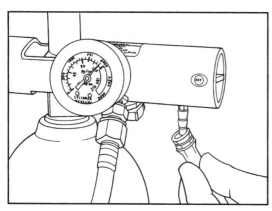

☐ **Attach the delivery device**

- ◆ Attach plastic tubing between flowmeter and delivery device.

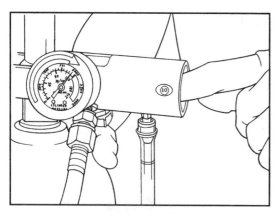

☐ **Adjust the flowmeter**

- ◆ Turn flowmeter to desired flow rate.

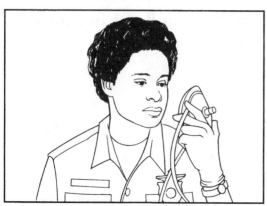

☐ **Verify oxygen flow**

- ◆ Listen and feel for oxygen flow through delivery device.

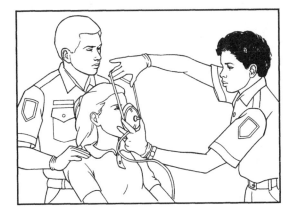

☐ **Place the delivery device on victim**

CAUTION: When breaking down the equipment, remove the delivery device from the victim's face, turn off the flowmeter, close the cylinder, then turn on the flowmeter to bleed the line. Finally, remove the regulator from the cylinder so other participant's may practice the complete skill.

Notes

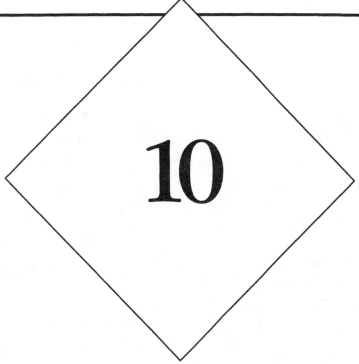

Cardiac Emergencies

◆ SUMMARY

It is important to recognize signs and symptoms that may indicate a heart attack. If you think someone is suffering from a heart attack or if you are unsure, summon more advanced medical personnel without delay. Provide care by helping the victim rest in the most comfortable position until help arrives.

When heartbeat and breathing stop, the condition is called cardiac arrest. A person who suffers a cardiac arrest is clinically dead, since no oxygen reaches the cells of vital organs. Irreversible brain damage will occur from lack of oxygen. By starting CPR immediately, you can help keep the brain supplied with oxygen. By summoning more advanced medical personnel, you can increase the cardiac arrest victim's chances for survival.

If the victim does not have a pulse, start CPR. Always remember these simple guidelines for CPR:

◆ Use the correct hand position.
◆ Compress down and up smoothly.
◆ Give 15 compressions in approximately 10 seconds.
◆ Give 2 slow breaths.
◆ Repeat this cycle of compressions and breaths 3 more times (4 times in all).
◆ Check for the return of a pulse.
◆ If there is no pulse, continue CPR, beginning with compressions.
◆ Check for the return of a pulse every few minutes.
◆ If the victim's pulse returns, stop CPR and check to see if the victim has started to breathe.
◆ If the victim is still not breathing, begin rescue breathing.

If two rescuers are available, begin two-rescuer CPR as soon as possible. If either rescuer tires, quickly change positions and continue. Once you start CPR, do not stop unnecessarily.

◆ OUTLINE

◆ LEARNING ACTIVITIES

Matching

Match each term with its definition. Write its letter on the line in front of the definition.

Terms

a. Cardiac arrest

b. Cardiovascular disease

c. Heart attack

d. Atherosclerosis

e. Cholesterol

f. Defibrillator

g. Coronary arteries

Definitions

1. _____ A sudden illness involving death of heart muscle tissue because of insufficient oxygen-rich blood reaching the cells

2. _____ A substance involved in coronary artery disease and found in certain foods, including egg yolks, and organ meats such as liver

3. _____ A chronic illness affecting the heart and blood vessels

4. _____ A condition in which the heart has stopped or beats too irregularly or weakly to pump blood

5. _____ The vessels that supply the heart muscles with oxygen-rich blood

6. _____ A buildup of fatty acids on the inner walls of the arteries

7. _____ A device that sends an electric shock to the heart to correct electrical abnormality

Match each compression/ventilation cycle with the correct type of CPR. Write its letter on the line in front of the type of CPR.

Compression/Ventilation Cycle

a. 5 compressions followed by 1 slow breath; 100 or more compressions per minute

b. 5 compressions followed by 1 slow breath; 80–100 compressions per minute

c. 15 compressions followed by 2 slow breaths; 80–100 compressions per minute

Type of CPR

1. _____ One-rescuer adult CPR

2. _____ Two-rescuer adult CPR

3. _____ Infant CPR

True/False

Circle T if the statement is true; circle F if it is false.

1. T F After doing 1 minute of CPR on an infant, you should check the brachial pulse for about 5 seconds.

2. T F An individual quits smoking after having smoked for 15 years. Over time, the person's risk of heart attack from smoking will decline until it becomes almost the same as for a person who has never smoked.

3. T F Brief, mild chest pain is usually a symptom of a heart attack.

4. T F Calling EMS personnel promptly is important in cases of cardiac arrest.

5. T F It is often difficult to find the correct hand position for chest compressions on an obese person because fat accumulates over the sternum.

6. T F You should stop providing CPR altogether if the victim vomits.

7. T F You should assist a victim complaining of chest pain in taking his or her prescribed medication if you are authorized to do so.

8. T F In two-rescuer CPR, the breath given after every fifth compression should be delivered without a pause in the compressions.

9. T F During one-rescuer CPR on an adult, you should relocate the correct hand position after each cycle of CPR.

10. T F Angina pectoris is a period of brief chest pain or pressure usually lasting less than 10 minutes and relieved by taking a prescribed medication.

11. T F Unconsciousness, absence of breathing, and absence of pulse are the primary signs of cardiac arrest.

12. T F If a victim has lost a significant amount of blood, the carotid pulse may not be found, even if effective chest compressions are being provided.

13. T F Routine exercise has been shown to decrease the risk of heart attack.

14. T F When a second rescuer becomes available to assist with CPR already in progress, he or she should immediately take over from the first rescuer.

15. T F Children do not often initially suffer a cardiac emergency.

16. T F Administration of oxygen by a trained person is appropriate emergency care for a victim experiencing chest pain or discomfort.

17. T F Your hand should be placed below the xiphoid process when performing CPR.

18. T F It is acceptable to stop CPR if you are too exhausted to continue.

19. T F CPR for a child is similar to an adult, in that it requires 15 compressions and 2 breaths.

20. T F The correct location for chest compressions on an infant is on the center of the sternum, just beneath the nipples.

Short Answer

Read each statement or question and write the correct answer or answers in the space provided.

1. What five key questions should you ask a victim about his or her chest pain?

2. What are seven circumstances in which it is appropriate to stop CPR after you have started?

3. Describe the four steps for locating and placing your hands in the correct position to provide chest compressions to an adult.

4. List three early signs and symptoms of a respiratory emergency in infants and children that could lead to a cardiac emergency.

5. In what three situations should you be able to perform two-rescuer CPR?

6. T F During CPR, you should remove your hand from the child's chest to deliver breaths and relocate your hand position when you return to the chest to deliver compressions.

◆ CASE STUDIES

Read the case studies and answer the questions that follow.

Case 10.1

You are called to the scene of a drowning. An 8-year-old child has just been removed from the water after being submerged for several minutes. The child is not breathing, and you feel no carotid pulse.

1. T F To avoid injuring the child, you should only perform rescue breathing.

2. To deliver chest compressions to this child, you would use the—

   a. Heel of one hand.

   b. Heel of two hands.

   c. Pads of two fingers.

   d. Pads of three fingers.

3. T F You should push the sternum of the child down from 1 to 1 1/2 inches with each chest compression.

4. T F Chest compressions should be delivered at a rate of 80–100 times per minute.

5. After you have started chest compressions, how often should you recheck this child's pulse?

Case 10.2

You are attending an office meeting at which a co-worker is giving a presentation. She suddenly stops and complains of chest pain and shortness of breath. She looks pale and is sweating.

1. Which step would you take first in caring for this victim?

   a. Have her stop her presentation and sit down.

   b. Call for an ambulance.

   c. Turn on the air conditioning.

   d. Have her lie on the floor and cover her with a blanket to prevent chilling.

2. T F With these signs and symptoms, it is unlikely that this individual is experiencing a heart attack.

3. Describe five actions you would take for this victim while waiting for advanced medical personnel to arrive.

4. If the victim is experiencing a heart attack, why is it very important for advanced medical personnel to arrive quickly?

5. Describe the cycle of chest compressions and ventilations when giving CPR to an infant.

Case 10.3

You rescue a six-month-old from an apartment fire. When you look, listen, and feel for breathing, you find that her breathing has stopped.

1. What will you do next in providing emergency care?

   a. Check for a pulse.

   b. Deliver two slow breaths.

   c. Do a finger sweep.

   d. Turn the infant over and deliver 5 back blows.

2. Where will you check this infant's pulse?

   a. At the carotid artery in the neck

   b. At the heart at the left nipple

   c. At the brachial artery in the arm

   d. At the radial artery in the wrist

3. Describe the correct hand position to give chest compressions to this infant.

4. T F While providing CPR to this infant, you should keep one hand on the victim's forehead to keep the airway open, while compressing the chest with 2 fingers of the other hand.

◆ SELF-ASSESSMENT

Circle the letter of the best answer.

1. The purpose of cardiopulmonary resuscitation (CPR) is to—

   a. Keep the brain supplied with oxygen until the heart can be restarted.

   b. Prevent clinical death from occurring in a victim of cardiac arrest.

   c. Restart heartbeat and breathing in a victim of cardiac arrest.

   d. All of the above.

2. The most common cause(s) of cardiac emergencies in children is/are—

   a. Poisoning.

   b. Near-drowning.

   c. Motor vehicle injury.

   d. Respiratory problems

3. What should you do if a victim's breathing and heartbeat return while you are giving CPR?

   a. Have a bystander transport you and the victim to the nearest hospital.

   b. Continue rescue breathing while waiting for advanced medical personnel to arrive.

   c. Complete a secondary survey before calling advanced medical personnel for assistance.

   d. Keep the airway open and monitor vital signs until advanced medical personnel arrive.

4. During two-rescuer CPR, the person giving the breaths should—

   a. Count aloud to keep the person giving the compressions at the proper rate.

   b. Periodically check the effectiveness of the compressions by checking the carotid pulse during CPR.

   c. Call for a stop in the compressions after every minute to check for a return of pulse.

   d. All of the above.

5. The most prominent sign(s) of a heart attack is/are—

   a. Difficulty breathing.

   b. Jaw and left arm pain.

   c. Nausea and sweating.

   d. Persistent chest pain.

6. In what position should you place a victim who may be experiencing a heart attack?

   a. The most comfortable position for the victim

   b. Sitting or semi-sitting

   c. Lying on the left side

   d. Lying on the back with legs elevated

7. High blood pressure can be controlled by—

   a. Losing excess weight.

   b. Changing dietary habits.

   c. Taking prescribed medication.

   d. All of the above.

8. Where should you place your hands to deliver effective chest compressions?

   a. Over the xiphoid process

   b. Over the lower half of the sternum

   c. On the middle of the sternum

   d. Just below the notch at the top of the sternum

9. Which is the primary sign of cardiac arrest?

   a. No breathing

   b. Absence of blood pressure

   c. Absence of a carotid pulse

   d. Dilation of the pupils

10. To deliver chest compressions on a child, you would use the—

    a. Heel of one hand.

    b. Pads of two fingers.

    c. Heel of two hands.

    d. Pads of three fingers.

Notes

Notes

PRACTICE SESSION: *CPR for an Adult*

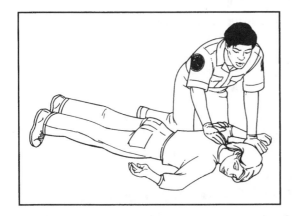

☐ Check for consciousness

- ◆ Tap and gently shake person.
- ◆ Shout, "Are you OK?"

If person does not respond...

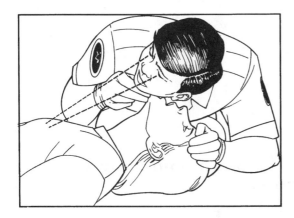

☐ Check for breathing

- ◆ Look, listen, and feel for about 5 seconds

If not breathing or you cannot tell...

- ◆ Position victim onto back while supporting the head and neck.
- ◆ Open the airway.
- ◆ Tilt head back and lift chin.
- ◆ Recheck breathing.
- ◆ Look, listen, and feel for about 5 seconds.

If person is not breathing...

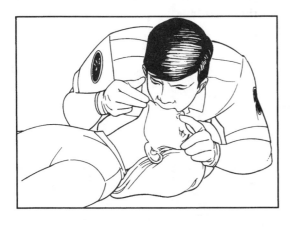

- ◆ Keep head tilted back.
- ◆ Pinch nose shut.
- ◆ Seal your lips tightly around person's mouth.
- ◆ Give 2 slow breaths, each lasting about 1 1/2 seconds.
- ◆ Watch to see that the breaths go in.

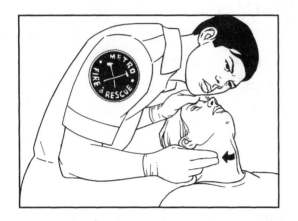

☐ Check for pulse

- ◆ Locate Adam's apple.
- ◆ Slide fingers down into groove of neck on side closer to you.
- ◆ Feel for pulse for 5 to 10 seconds.

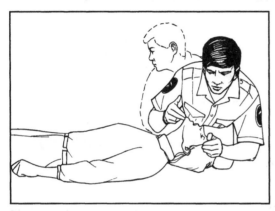

☐ Check for severe bleeding

- ◆ Look from head to toe for severe bleeding.

If person does not have a pulse...

- ◆ **Begin CPR.**

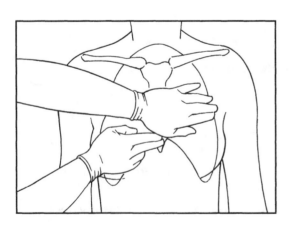

☐ Find hand position

- ◆ Locate notch at lower end of sternum.
- ◆ Place heel of other hand on sternum next to fingers.
- ◆ Remove hand from notch and put it on top of other hand.
- ◆ Keep fingers off chest.

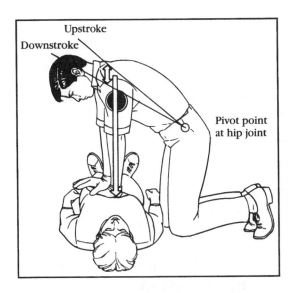

☐ Give 15 compressions

- ◆ Position shoulders over hands.
- ◆ Compress sternum 1 1/2 to 2 inches.
- ◆ Do 15 compressions in about 10 seconds.
- ◆ Compress down and up smoothly, keeping hand contact with chest at all times.

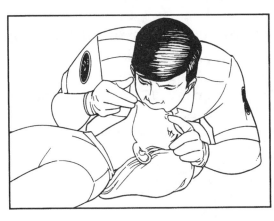

☐ Give 2 slow breaths

- ◆ Open airway with head-tilt/chin-lift.
- ◆ Pinch nose shut and seal your lips tightly around person's mouth.
- ◆ Give 2 slow breaths, each lasting about 1 1/2 seconds.
- ◆ Watch chest to see that your breaths go in.

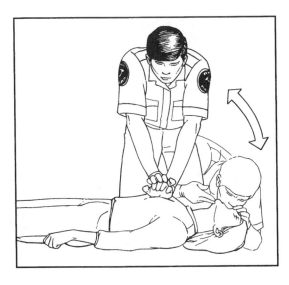

☐ Repeat compression/breathing cycles

- ◆ Repeat cycles of 15 compressions and 2 breaths.

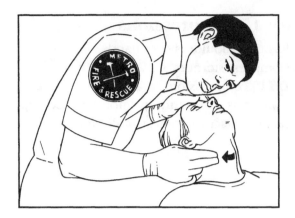

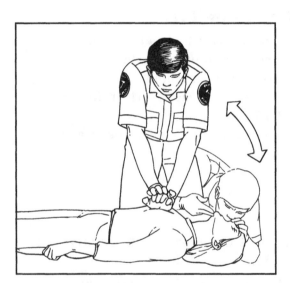

☐ **Recheck pulse**

- ◆ After about 1 minute, feel for pulse for about 5 seconds.

If person has a pulse and is breathing...

- ◆ Keep airway open.
- ◆ Monitor breathing.

If person has a pulse but is still not breathing...

- ◆ Do rescue breathing.

If person does not have a pulse and is not breathing...

☐ **Continue compression/breathing cycles**

- ◆ Locate correct hand position.
- ◆ Continue cycles of 15 compressions and 2 slow breaths.
- ◆ Recheck pulse every few minutes.

PRACTICE SESSION: *CPR for a Child*

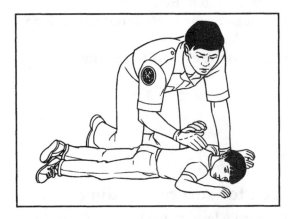

☐ Check for consciousness

- ◆ Tap and gently shake child's shoulder.

If child does not respond...

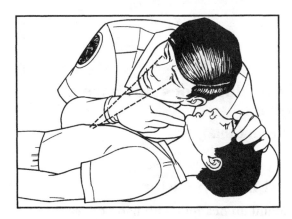

☐ Check for breathing

- ◆ Look, listen, and feel for about 5 seconds.

If not breathing or you cannot tell...

- ◆ Position victim onto back while supporting the head and neck.
- ◆ Open the airway.
- ◆ Tilt head back and lift chin.
- ◆ Recheck breathing.
- ◆ Look, listen, and feel for about 5 seconds.

If child is not breathing...

- ◆ Keep head tilted back.
- ◆ Seal your lips tightly around child's mouth and nose.
- ◆ Give 2 slow breaths, each lasting about 1 1/2 seconds.
- ◆ Watch to see that the breaths go in.

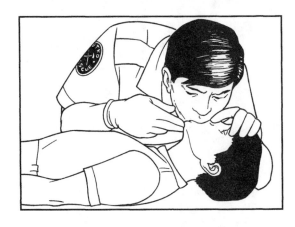

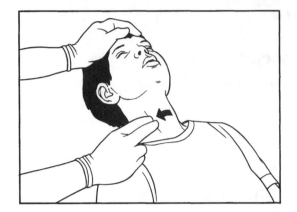

☐ Check for pulse

- ◆ Locate carotid pulse.
- ◆ Slide fingers down into groove of neck on side closer to you.
- ◆ Feel for pulse for 5 to 10 seconds.

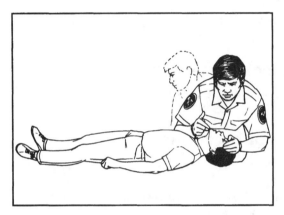

☐ Check for severe bleeding

- ◆ Look from head to toe for severe bleeding.

If the child does not have a pulse...

- ◆ **Begin CPR.**

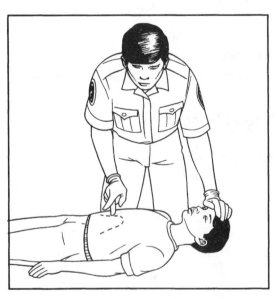

☐ Find hand position

- ◆ Maintain head-tilt with hand on forehead.
- ◆ Locate notch at lower end of sternum with other hand.

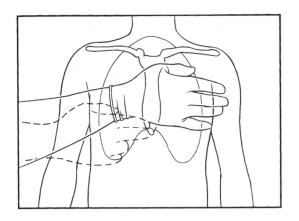

♦ Place heel of same hand on sternum immediately above where fingers were placed.

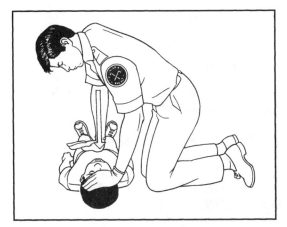

☐ Give 5 compressions

♦ Position shoulders over hands.
♦ Compress sternum 1 to 1 1/2 inches.
♦ Do 5 compressions in about 3 seconds.
♦ Compress down and up smoothly, keeping hand contact with chest at all times.
♦ Maintain head-tilt with hand on forehead.

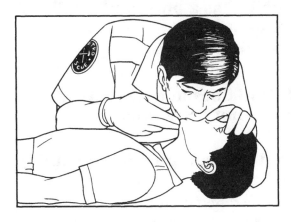

☐ Give 1 slow breath

♦ Open airway with head-tilt/chin-lift.
♦ Pinch nose shut and seal your lips tightly around child's mouth.
♦ Give 1 slow breath lasting about 1 1/2 seconds.
♦ Watch chest to see that your breath goes in.

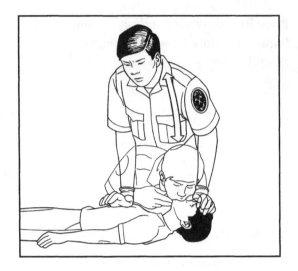

☐ **Repeat compression/breathing cycles**

   ◆ Repeat cycles of 5 compressions and 1 breath.

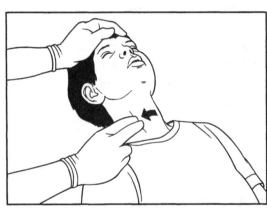

☐ **Recheck pulse**

   ◆ After about 1 minute, feel for pulse for about 5 seconds.

If child has a pulse and is breathing...

   ◆ **Keep airway open.**
   ◆ **Monitor breathing.**

If child has a pulse but is still not breathing...

   ◆ **Do rescue breathing.**

If child does not have a pulse and is not breathing...

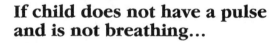

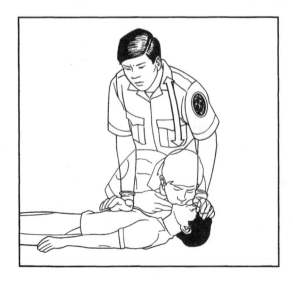

☐ **Continue compression/breathing cycles**

   ◆ Locate correct hand position.
   ◆ Continue cycles of 5 compressions and 1 breath.
   ◆ Recheck pulse every few minutes.

PRACTICE SESSION: *CPR for an Infant*

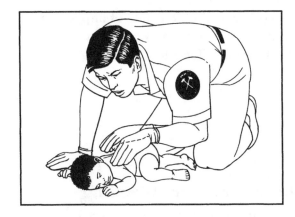

□ **Check for consciousness**

- ◆ Tap and gently shake infant's shoulder.

If infant does not respond...

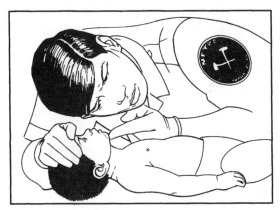

□ **Check for breathing**

- ◆ Look, listen, and feel for about 5 seconds.

If not breathing or you cannot tell...

- ◆ Position victim onto back while supporting the head and neck.
- ◆ Open the airway.
- ◆ Tilt head back and lift chin.
- ◆ Recheck breathing.
- ◆ Look, listen, and feel for about 5 seconds.

If infant is not breathing...

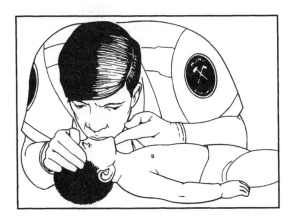

- ◆ Keep head tilted back.
- ◆ Seal your lips tightly around infant's mouth and nose.
- ◆ Give 2 slow breaths, each lasting about 1 1/2 seconds.
- ◆ Watch to see that the breaths go in.

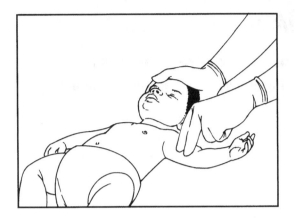

☐ Check for pulse

- ◆ Locate brachial pulse.
- ◆ Place fingers on the inside of upper arm midway between elbow and shoulder.
- ◆ Feel for pulse for 5 to 10 seconds.

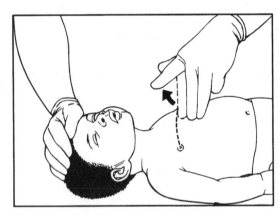

☐ Check for severe bleeding

- ◆ Look from head to toe for severe bleeding.

If infant does not have a pulse...

- ◆ **Begin CPR.**

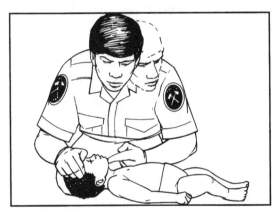

☐ Find hand position

- ◆ Maintain head-tilt with hand on forehead.
- ◆ Place pads of fingers next to imaginary line running across chest connecting nipples.
- ◆ Raise your index finger.
- ◆ Adjust finger position if necessary.

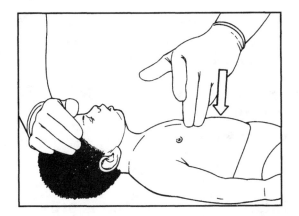

☐ Give 5 compressions

- ◆ Position hand over fingers.
- ◆ Compress sternum 1/2 to 1 inch.
- ◆ Do 5 compressions in about 3 seconds.
- ◆ Compress down and up smoothly, keeping finger in contact with chest at all times.
- ◆ Maintain head-tilt with hand on forehead.

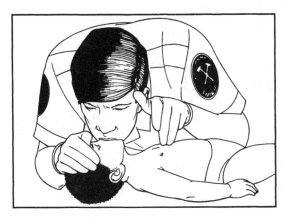

☐ Give 1 slow breath

- ◆ Maintain finger contact with chest.
- ◆ Seal your lips tightly around infant's mouth and nose.
- ◆ Give 1 slow breath lasting about 1 1/2 seconds.
- ◆ Watch chest to see that your breath goes in.

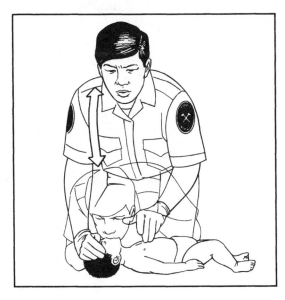

☐ Repeat compression/breathing cycles

- ◆ Repeat cycles of 5 compressions and 1 breath.

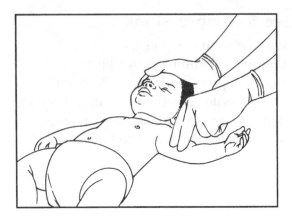

☐ **Recheck pulse**

- ♦ After about 1 minute, feel for brachial pulse for about 5 seconds.

If infant has a pulse and is breathing...

- ♦ **Keep airway open.**
- ♦ **Monitor breathing.**
- ♦ **Wait for EMS personnel to arrive.**

If infant has a pulse but is still not breathing...

- ♦ **Do rescue breathing.**

If infant does not have a pulse and is not breathing...

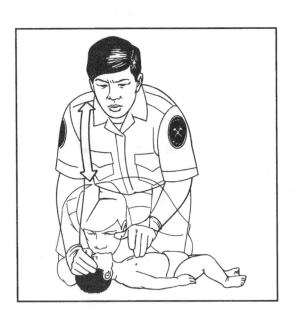

☐ **Continue compression/breathing cycles**

- ♦ Locate correct compression position.
- ♦ Continue cycles of 5 compressions and 1 breath.
- ♦ Recheck pulse every few minutes.

PRACTICE SESSION: *Two-Rescuer CPR—Beginning CPR Together*

☐ **Ventilator—Complete primary survey**

♦ Check for consciousness.
♦ Position the person.

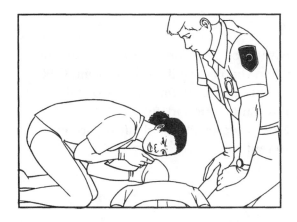

♦ Open airway and check for breathing.

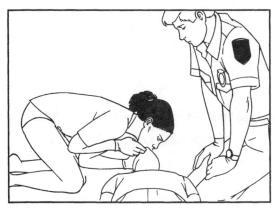

♦ Give 2 slow breaths.

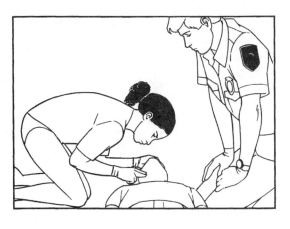

♦ Check for pulse. Say, "No pulse."

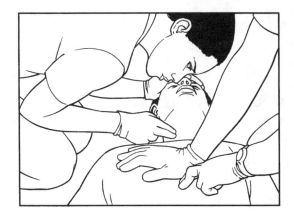

☐ Compressor—Find hand position and give 5 compressions

- ◆ Locate hand position while ventilator checks pulse.

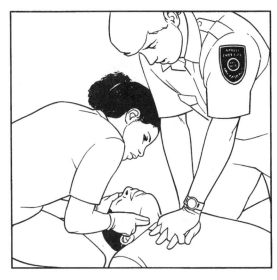

- ◆ Give 5 compressions in about 4 seconds, when ventilator tells you to "Begin CPR."
- ◆ Count out loud, "One-and, two-and, three-and, four-and, five."
- ◆ Stop compressions and allow partner to ventilate.

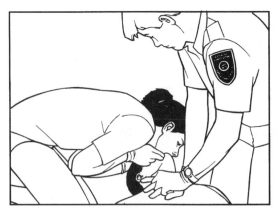

☐ Ventilator—Give 1 slow breath

- ◆ Give 1 slow breath, lasting about 1 1/2 seconds.

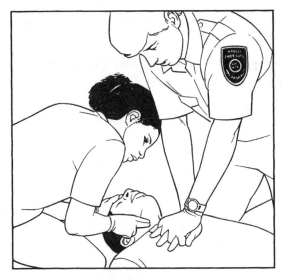

☐ **Both rescuers—Continue CPR**

- ◆ Repeat cycles of 5 compressions and 1 breath.
- ◆ Ventilator—periodically check compression effectiveness by checking pulse while partner is giving compressions.

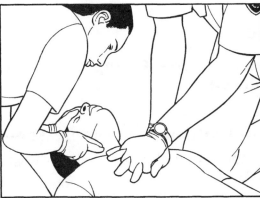

☐ **Recheck pulse and breathing**

- ◆ At end of first minute, check pulse for about 5 seconds.

If person has a pulse...

- ◆ **Recheck breathing.**
- ◆ **If person is not breathing, do rescue breathing.**
- ◆ **Recheck pulse every minute.**

If person does not have a pulse...

- ◆ **Say, "No pulse, continue CPR."**
- ◆ **Continue CPR.**
- ◆ **Recheck pulse every few minutes.**

PRACTICE SESSION: *Two-Rescuer CPR—Changing Positions*

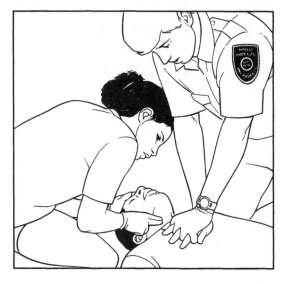

☐ **Compressor—Call for position change**

- ◆ Say, "Change-and, two-and, three-and, four-and, five."

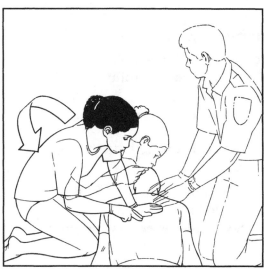

☐ **Both rescuers—Change positions**

From Ventilator to Compressor—

- ◆ Complete 1 slow breath at end of "change" cycle.
- ◆ Move quickly to person's chest.
- ◆ Find hand position. Wait for signal to begin compressions.

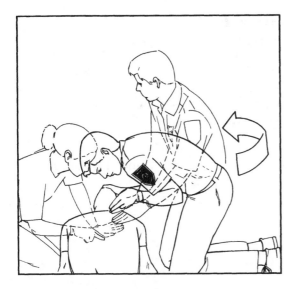

From compressor to ventilator—

- ◆ Complete compression cycle.
- ◆ Move quickly to person's head and become ventilator.
- ◆ Feel for pulse for about 5 seconds.
- ◆ Say, "No pulse, continue CPR."

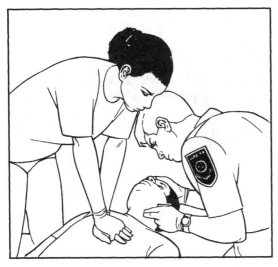

☐ Both rescuers—Continue CPR

- ◆ New compressor begins compressions.
- ◆ Both rescuers continue CPR with cycles of 5 compressions and 1 breath.
- ◆ New ventilator periodically checks for effectiveness of compressions and rechecks pulse and breathing every few minutes.

PRACTICE SESSION: *Entry of a Second Rescuer When*
One-Rescuer CPR is in Progress
(Optional practice session)

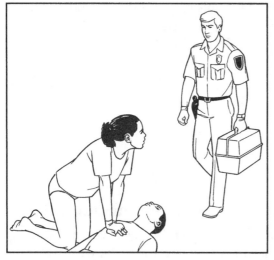

☐ **Second rescuer—Identify**
yourself

- ◆ Identify yourself.
- ◆ Determine if more advanced medical
  personnel have been called.

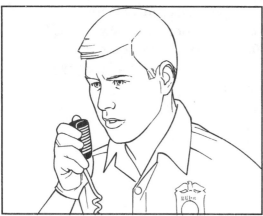

☐ **Summon advanced medical**
personnel (if necessary)

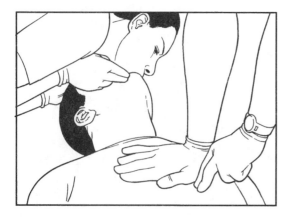

☐ **Get into position to give**
compressions

- ◆ Position yourself by person's chest as
  first rescuer completes full cycle of 15
  compressions and 2 breaths.
- ◆ Locate hand position.

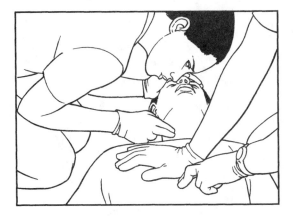

☐ **First rescuer—Check pulse**

- ◆ Complete compression/ventilation cycle.
- ◆ Say, "Pulse check," and feel for carotid pulse for about 5 seconds.
- ◆ If no pulse, say, "No pulse, continue CPR."

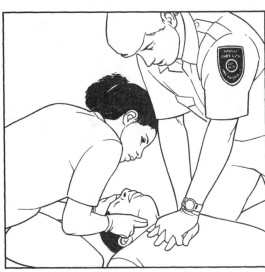

☐ **Both rescuers—Continue CPR**

- ◆ Second rescuer begins compressions.
- ◆ First rescuer gives 1 breath after each set of 5 compressions.
- ◆ First rescuer periodically checks for effectiveness of compressions and rechecks pulse and breathing every few minutes.

Notes

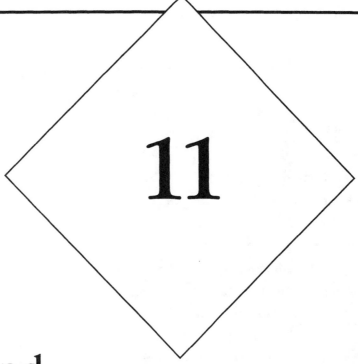

Bleeding and Shock

◆ SUMMARY

One of the most important things you can do in any emergency is to recognize and control severe bleeding. External bleeding is easily recognized and should be cared for immediately. Check and care for severe bleeding during the initial assessment. Severe external bleeding is life threatening. Although internal bleeding is less obvious, it also can be life threatening. Recognize when a serious injury has occurred and suspect internal bleeding. You may not identify internal bleeding until you perform the physical exam and history. When you identify or suspect severe bleeding, request an ambulance so that the victim can be transported quickly to a hospital. Continue to provide care until more advanced medical personnel arrive and take over.

Do not wait for shock to develop before providing care to a victim of injury or sudden illness. Care for life-threatening conditions, such as breathing problems or severe external bleeding, before caring for lesser injuries. Remember that managing shock effectively begins with recognizing a situation in which shock may develop and giving appropriate care. Shock is a factor in serious injuries and illnesses, particularly if there is blood loss or if the normal function of the heart is interrupted. With serious injuries or illnesses, shock is often the final stage before death. You cannot always prevent shock by giving emergency care, but you can usually slow its progress. Summon more advanced medical personnel immediately if you notice signs and symptoms of shock. Shock can often be reversed by advanced medical care, but only if the victim is reached in time.

◆ OUTLINE

◆ LEARNING ACTIVITIES

Matching

Match each term with its definition. Write its letter on the line in front of the definition.

Terms

a. Blood volume

b. Platelets

c. External bleeding

d. Internal bleeding

e. Arteries

f. Red blood cells

g. Hemorrhage

h. White blood cells

i. Vital organs

j. Shock

Definitions

1. _____ Blood cell fragments that aid in clotting

2. _____ A component of blood that produces antibodies

3. _____ The vessels carrying blood away from the heart

4. _____ A component of blood produced in the marrow of large bones

5. _____ The rapid loss of a large amount of blood

6. _____ Blood loss such as from a cut finger

7. _____ The total amount of blood circulating in the body

8. _____ Blood loss such as occurs from a ruptured spleen

9. _____ A condition in which the circulatory system fails to adequately circulate oxygen-rich blood to all parts of the body

10. _____ Structures, such as the heart, lungs, and brain, with functions that are essential to life

True/False

Circle T if the statement is true; circle F if it is false.

1. T F You can control serious internal bleeding by applying ice packs to the injured area.

2. T F When trying to control external bleeding, leave blood-soaked dressings in place.

3. T F Capillaries are very small blood vessels in which the exchange of oxygen and waste products between the blood and body cells takes place.

4. T F Blood that oozes from a wound is a sign of severe external bleeding.

5. T F One function of blood is to help maintain constant body temperature.

6. T F When bleeding occurs, the body begins to compensate for the blood loss by diverting oxygen-rich blood to the vital organs.

7. T F An increase in blood pressure is a sign of significant internal blood loss.

8. T F A pressure point is a site on the body where pressure can be applied to a major artery to slow the flow of blood to a body part.

9. T F Capillary bleeding is the loss of a large amount of blood in a short time.

10. T F In controlling external bleeding, the injured area should be lowered below the level of the heart.

11. T F Discoloration of the skin in the injured area is a sign of internal bleeding.

12. T F If you wore gloves while applying direct pressure to a bleeding wound and the gloves were not punctured or torn, it would not be necessary to wash your hands after providing care.

13. T F Applying pressure at a pressure point is the first step in controlling external bleeding.

14. T F If a victim of serious injury complains of extreme thirst, you should provide water to help minimize shock.

15. T F Shock is a condition resulting only from severe blood loss.

16. T F Because the body responds to shock by reducing the amount of blood going to the skin, a victim in shock appears pale and feels cool.

17. T F A slow and strong pulse, rapid breathing, and nausea, are signs and symptoms of shock.

18. T F An individual who is injured and frightened is less likely to develop shock than one who is calm.

19. T F Having an adequate amount of blood circulating in the body is one of the conditions necessary to avoid shock.

Short Answer

Read each statement and write the correct answer or answers in the space provided.

1. List the three major functions of blood.

2. What are the two key signs of severe external bleeding?

3. List at least five signs and symptoms of severe internal bleeding.

4. List in order the steps for controlling external bleeding.

5. What is one of the most common early indications of shock?

6. List five things you can do to care for shock.

7. List the three conditions necessary to maintain adequate blood flow.

◆ CASE STUDIES

Read the case studies and answer the questions that follow.

Case 11.1

You arrive at the scene of a motor vehicle crash. The driver has already gotten out of the car and is sitting on the ground near the road. He complains of pain in his abdomen and says he feels nauseated from hitting the steering wheel. When you look under his shirt, you see that the skin across the lower abdomen is bruised. He says his abdomen is tender to your touch. As you are talking to the victim, a second motorist stops and offers to help.

1. Which should you do in caring for this victim?

   a. Administer oxygen if it is available and you are trained to do so.

   b. Reassure the victim.

   c. Summon more advanced medical personnel.

   d. All of the above.

2. T   F   This victim should be kept in a sitting position to protect his airway in case he vomits.

3. Describe the guidelines for the care you will give this victim.

Case 11.2

You respond to a call from a parent at a farm where a child's arm has been injured in machinery. Her forearm is deeply lacerated and bleeding heavily.

1. T F   You should put on gloves before applying direct pressure to the wound.

2. Which of the following would you do as part of your care for this child?

    a. Apply a pressure bandage to the wound.

    b. Administer supplemental oxygen to the victim.

    c. Apply additional dressings if the first one becomes soaked with blood.

    d. All of the above.

3. If a pressure bandage does not control the bleeding from the forearm, which pressure point should you use to slow the bleeding?

    a. Brachial

    b. Femoral

    c. Axillary

    d. Carotid

Case 11.3

A 35-year-old man has fallen 7 feet from a ladder in a warehouse. You find him lying on his back on the cement floor. He is complaining about pain in his leg and hip.

1. You check his pulse and find it to be weak and at a rate of 120. What does this probably indicate?

    a. He may be losing blood internally.

    b. He has been badly frightened by the accident.

    c. His heart is compensating for a loss of blood internally by beating faster.

    d. All of the above.

2. As you check the rest of the man's vital signs, you notice that his skin is moist, cool, and a little pale. He complains of "feeling lightheaded." What do these signs mean to you?

    a. Moist skin is a normal stress reaction to injury.

    b. The patient's body is trying to compensate for serious injury.

    c. It is normal for someone in this situation to be a little confused and scared.

    d. The patient is recovering from the situation, as he is quieter and seems to be calming down.

3. While you wait for advanced medical personnel to arrive, the victim's condition continues to deteriorate. His breathing rate is fast, pulse is fast but weak, and he is responsive only to painful stimuli. What should you do now?

    a. Maintain an adequate airway and give oxygen if available.

    b. Cover him to prevent chilling.

    c. Elevate his hips and legs.

    d. a and b.

◆ SELF-ASSESSMENT

Circle the letter of the best answer.

1. The term used to indicate the loss of a large amount of blood in a short time is—

    a. Evisceration.

    b. Hemorrhage.

    c. Internal bleeding.

    d. Capillary bleeding.

2. One of the major functions of blood is to—

   a. Transmit impulses to the brain.

   b. Prevent internal bleeding.

   c. Transport nutrients and oxygen to the cells.

   d. Maintain pressure within blood vessels.

3. Why might severe bleeding result in death?

   a. The supply of necessary nutrients to the heart is reduced.

   b. Decreased blood volume deprives body tissues of oxygen.

   c. Severe blood loss results in kidney failure and death.

   d. Blood vessels collapse as blood volume decreases.

4. The methods used to control external bleeding include—

   a. Indirect pressure, pressure bandage, and venous pressure.

   b. Direct pressure, pressure wrap, and venous pressure point.

   c. Indirect pressure, pressure wrap, and arterial pressure point.

   d. Direct pressure, pressure bandage, and arterial pressure point.

5. Signs of minor internal bleeding from capillaries beneath the skin of the forearm include—

   a. Bruising.

   b. Drop in blood pressure.

   c. Cool, moist skin.

   d. All of the above.

6. Care for severe internal bleeding includes—

   a. Immediately summoning more advanced medical personnel.

   b. Protecting the victim against chilling.

   c. Administering supplemental oxygen if it is available and you are trained to do so.

   d. All of the above.

7. Which of the following measures would minimize shock?

   a. Cooling the victim's body

   b. Warming the victim's body

   c. Keeping the victim from getting chilled or overheated

   d. Allowing the victim's body temperature to regulate itself

8. The appropriate position for a victim who is showing signs of shock as a result of injuries to the head and neck would be—

   a. Lying flat on the back.

   b. Legs elevated about 12 inches.

   c. On the side with the head slightly elevated.

   d. Head and shoulders elevated about 12 inches.

9. What can cause a victim to develop shock?

   a. Severe blood loss

   b. Too little oxygen in the bloodstream

   c. Injury to the spinal cord

   d. All of the above

10. The skin of a victim in shock appears pale and feels cool because—

    a. Shock damages the temperature control centers in the brain and spinal cord.

    b. The body responds to shock by constricting blood vessels in the arms, legs, and skin.

    c. Shock causes the heart to beat more slowly, reducing the amount of heat generated by the body.

    d. The body responds to shock by cooling itself to decrease energy needs.

11. If you suspect possible head, neck or back injuries, you should avoid—

    a. Administering oxygen.

    b. Elevating the legs.

    c. Controlling external bleeding.

    d. Caring for airway and breathing problems.

12. Three things you can do to minimize shock are to —

    a. Splint fractures, keep the victim warm, and start an IV.

    b. Administer oxygen if it is available and you are trained to do so, splint fractures, elevate the victim's head.

    c. Elevate the victim's legs, prevent chilling, and start an IV.

    d. Prevent chilling, administer oxygen if it is available and you are trained to do so, and elevate the victim's legs.

Notes

Notes

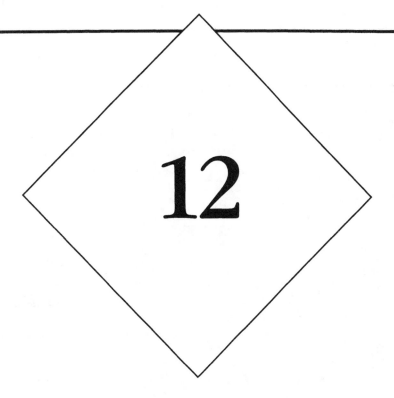

Specific Injuries

◆ SUMMARY

Caring for wounds is not difficult. You need only follow the basic guidelines to control bleeding and minimize the risk of infection. Remember that with minor wounds, your primary concern is to cleanse the wound to prevent infection. With major wounds, you should control the bleeding quickly using direct pressure and elevation and summon more advanced medical professionals. Dressings and bandages, when correctly applied, help control bleeding, reduce pain, and can minimize the danger of infection.

Burn injuries damage the layers of the skin and sometimes the internal structures, as well. Heat, chemicals, electricity, and radiation all cause burns. When caring for a burn victim, always first ensure your personal safety. When the scene is safe, approach the victim and do an initial assessment and a physical examination if necessary.

Once the victim has been removed from the burn source, follow the steps of burn care:
◆ Cool the burned area with water to minimize additional tissue destruction.
◆ Keep air away from the burned area by covering it with dry, sterile dressings, clean sheets, or other cloth.
◆ Keep the victim from getting chilled or overheated to minimize shock.
◆ Summon more advanced medical personnel for any critical burn.

In addition, always check for inhalation injury if the person has a heat or chemical burn involving the face. With electrical burns, check carefully for other problems, such as difficulty breathing, cardiac problems, and painful, swollen deformed areas.

◆ OUTLINE

Any items marked with ** indicate information found only in the Enrichment section of the text.

◆ LEARNING ACTIVITIES

Matching

Match each term with its definition. Write its letter on the line in front of the definition.

Terms

a. Abrasion

b. Occlusive dressing

c. Layer of fat

d. Full-thickness burn

e. Dermis

f. Avulsion

g. Soft tissue

h. Superficial burn

i. Dressing

j. Laceration

k. Puncture

l. Bandage

m. Critical burn

n. Embedded object

Definitions

1. _____ The layer of the skin containing nerves and sweat glands

2. _____ Material used to hold a splint or wound covering in place

3. _____ Any burn that is potentially life threatening, disabling, or disfiguring

4. _____ A burn injury that involves only the epidermis

5. _____ An injury created when the skin is pierced with a pointed object

6. _____ A burn injury involving both layers of skin and underlying tissues

7. _____ An injury in which a portion of the skin is partially torn away and hangs like a flap

8. _____ Body structures including the layers of skin, fat, and muscles

9. _____ An open wound in which the skin has been rubbed or scraped away

10. _____ A structure that lies beneath the skin and helps maintain body temperature

11. _____ A specialized covering that does not allow air to pass through it

12. _____ A cut with jagged or smooth edges, caused by a sharp object

13. _____ Material placed directly over a wound to absorb blood and prevent infection

14. _____ An object that remains in an open wound

True/False

Circle T if the statement is true; circle F if it is false.

1. T F Full-thickness burns are less likely to cause shock than partial-thickness burns because full-thickness burns can be relatively painless and partial-thickness burns cause severe pain.

2. T F The difference between a dressing and a bandage is that a dressing is applied directly over an open wound and a bandage is used to hold a dressing in place.

3. T F If no sterile dressing is available to place over a severely bleeding wound, the next best thing to use to control the bleeding is your bare hand.

4. T F Emergency care for a sunburn that involves multiple layers of skin includes application of ointments made specially to reduce the effects of sunburn.

5. T F Swelling and bruising are signs of a closed wound.

6. T F The best initial defense against infection of an open wound is to thoroughly cleanse it with alcohol.

7. T F The skin of a victim with a partial-thickness burn will usually be red and dry.

8. T F You should summon more advanced medical personnel for a child who has suffered partial-thickness burns.

9. T F A victim with a full-thickness burn may develop the signs and symptoms of shock from loss of body fluids through the burn.

10. T F If glass is embedded in a victim's upper arm, you should carefully remove the glass and apply direct pressure over the wound.

11. T F Bandages can be used to support an injured limb or body part.

12. T F A sucking chest wound should be cared for by applying an occlusive dressing.

13. T F Burns are a type of soft tissue injury primarily caused by heat.

14. T F More advanced medical personnel should be called immediately for an adult victim who has a superficial burn on the shoulder.

15. T F You should care for sunburn, as you would for any other burn.

16. T F The spleen is protected somewhat by the lower left ribs.

17. T F If, after you bandage a wound on the forearm, the fingers of the victim's hand become cool and pale, you should loosen the bandage slightly.

18. T F If abdominal organs protrude through a wound, you should replace them and apply a dressing and bandage securely over the wound to prevent infection.

**19. T F Injury is the leading cause of death among people ages 45 to 70.

**20. T F Injury is the most common cause of hospitalization among people under the age of 45.

Short Answer

Read each statement or question and write the correct answer or answers in the space provided.

1. Describe three steps in the care for a victim who has an embedded object in the leg.

2. What five conditions determine the severity of a burn?

3. What should you do to minimize shock in a victim of extensive burns?

4. What are the four main types of open wounds?

5. Describe six aspects of care for a major open wound.

◆ CASE STUDIES

Read the case studies and answer the questions that follow.

Case 12.1

You are working at a metal shop and are called to help an injured worker. The worker's left arm was caught in a cutting machine and has been completely severed (amputated) at the middle of the forearm. He is lying on the floor of the shop, conscious, and in severe pain.

1. T F Since the upper forearm has been completely severed, you can expect severe bleeding, which can probably be controlled by using a pressure point.

2. T F To minimize the danger of infection, wash the wound with water for a few seconds before controlling the bleeding.

3. Which of these measures should you take to minimize the danger of disease transmission?

   a. Wear a pair of disposable gloves while controlling bleeding and applying a bandage.

   b. Wear protective eyewear and a surgical mask while caring for the victim.

   c. Wash your hands after completing care and removing your gloves.

   d. a and c.

4. Which condition will the victim probably suffer shortly?

   a. Infection

   b. Respiratory shock

   c. Shock

   d. High blood pressure

Case 12.2

You are summoned to the scene of a fire. While you are preparing to enter the house, a woman runs out with her clothes on fire.

1. Which is your first step in responding to this victim?

   a. Do an initial assessment.

   b. Cool the burned area.

   c. Summon specially trained personnel.

   d. Extinguish the flames on the clothing.

2. You determine that the woman is conscious and able to talk. Parts of her dress are charred. She has partial-thickness burns on her left arm and back. How will you cool these burns? What will you not use to cool them?

3. T F You should carefully remove all pieces of charred clothing that are sticking to the woman's skin by gently washing the area to loosen the clothing.

4. The woman has partial-thickness burns covering her entire chest and back. You see no other burns during your physical exam. Using the Rule of Nines, identify what percentage of her body is burned?

   a. 9 percent

   b. 18 percent

   c. 27 percent

   d. 36 percent

5. T F This would be considered a critical burn, and advanced medical personnel should be called immediately.

6. What should you use to cover this woman's burns to keep out air and decrease pain?

   a. Moist, sterile dressings

   b. Dry, sterile dressings

   c. Sterile occlusive dressings

   d. Burn ointment and sterile dressings

Case Study 12.3

You are called to the scene of an industrial incident. A worker was injured when the compressed gas cylinder she was testing exploded. She is lying on the floor gasping for breath, and her lips look bluish. The left side of the front of her shirt is torn and soaked with blood. As she tries to speak to you, she coughs up blood.

1. As you assess the victim, you hear a gurgling sound from the left side of the rib cage each time she gasps for breath. You would immediately suspect that she has sustained a—

    a. Flail chest.

    b. Fractured sternum.

    c. Sucking chest wound.

    d. Penetrating abdominal wound.

2. T F Your immediate care for this injury is to immobilize the injured area of the rib cage to make it easier for the victim to breathe.

3. Which of the following would you use to cover the injury on the left side of the chest?

    a. Gauze pad

    b. Triangular bandage

    c. Universal dressing

    d. Occlusive dressing

◆ **SELF-ASSESSMENT**

Circle the letter of the best answer.

1. Which of the following describes skin that has been superficially burned?

    a. Red, dry, and painful

    b. Pale, wet, and painful

    c. Red, wet, and painless

    d. Mottled, dry, and painless

2. When bandaging a forearm, you should—

    a. Cover the hand and fingers loosely.

    b. Leave the fingers of the hand exposed.

    c. Wrap the hand and fingers tightly to prevent swelling.

    d. Place a rolled dressing in the palm of the hand, close the hand, and wrap it completely.

3. A woman has splashed paint remover into her eyes. What should you do?

    a. Flush her eyes with warm water for at least 10 minutes.

    b. Flush her eyes with vinegar and water to neutralize the chemical.

    c. Flush her eyes continuously with cool tap water until more advanced medical personnel arrive.

    d. Flush her eyes with water for 2 to 3 minutes and call more advanced medical personnel.

4. A wound in which the skin is not broken and the area discolors and swells is a(n)—

    a. Closed wound.

    b. Open wound.

    c. Superficial burn.

    d. Avulsion.

5. In which of the following situations should you immediately call for more advanced medical personnel?

    a. A partial-thickness water scald to the arm of a 30-year-old man

    b. A blistering grease burn on the arm of a 68-year-old woman

    c. A partial-thickness sunburn on the back of a 26-year-old woman

    d. All of the above

6. When a burn appears brown or charred, shows white tissue underneath, and is almost painless, which layer(s) of soft tissue have been injured?

   a. The epidermis

   b. The epidermis and dermis

   c. The epidermis, dermis, and fatty tissues

   d. The epidermis, dermis, and underlying soft tissue structures

7. How would you minimize the risk of infection in a minor abrasion?

   a. Wash the abrasion with soap and water.

   b. Clean the area with hydrogen peroxide or alcohol.

   c. Take the victim to a doctor for a tetanus booster.

   d. All of the above.

8. Which purposes do bandages serve?

   a. Provide a sterile covering for wounds and control bleeding.

   b. Apply pressure to control bleeding and provide support to injured body parts.

   c. Reduce pain in open wounds and hold dressings in place.

   d. Prevent air from reaching a wound and apply ointments.

9. How would you care for a wound with minimal bleeding and superficial damage?

   a. Wash the wound with soap and water before controlling bleeding.

   b. After bleeding is stopped, apply an antibiotic ointment if one is available.

   c. Apply a sterile dressing over the wound and then apply a bandage.

   d. All of the above.

10. In treating the victim of an electrical injury, you should—

    a. Push the victim away from the electrical wires with a dry pole or stick.

    b. Cover any burns with a dry, sterile dressing.

    c. Look for an entrance and an exit wound.

    d. b and c.

Notes

PRACTICE SESSION: *Care for a Major Open Wound (Forearm)*

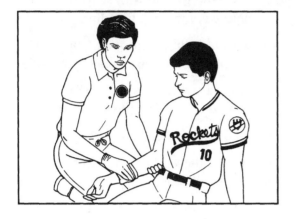

☐ **Apply direct pressure**

◆ Place sterile dressings or clean cloth over wound.

◆ Press firmly against wound with your hand.

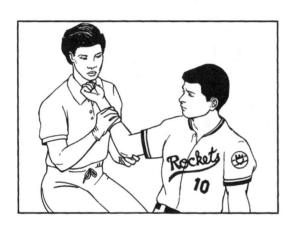

☐ **Elevate the body part**

◆ Raise wound above level of heart if possible.

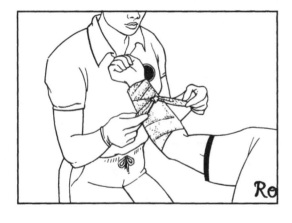

☐ **Apply a pressure bandage**

◆ Using a roller bandage, cover dressing completely, using overlapping turns.

◆ Secure the bandage.

◆ If blood soaks through the bandage, place additional dressings and bandages over the wound.

If bleeding stops...

◆ Determine if further care is needed.

If bleeding does not stop...

◆ Summon more advanced emergency personnel.

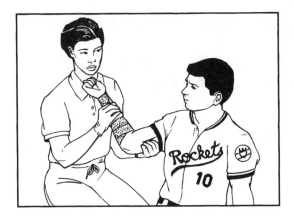

☐ Use a pressure point

- ◆ Maintain direct pressure and elevation.
- ◆ Locate brachial artery.
- ◆ Press the brachial artery against the underlying bone.

Continue to take steps to minimize shock

- ◆ Maintain direct pressure, elevation, and pressure point.
- ◆ Position person on back.
- ◆ Monitor ABCs.
- ◆ Maintain normal body temperature.
- ◆ Apply additional dressings and/or bandages as necessary.

PRACTICE SESSION: *Care for a Major Open Wound (Leg)*

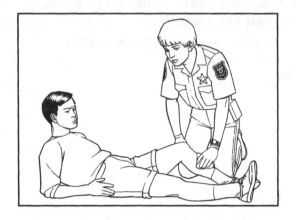

☐ **Apply direct pressure**

♦ Place sterile dressing or clean cloth over wound.

♦ Press firmly against wound with your hand.

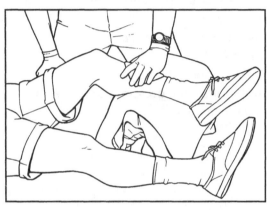

☐ **Elevate the body part**

♦ Raise wound above level of heart, if possible.

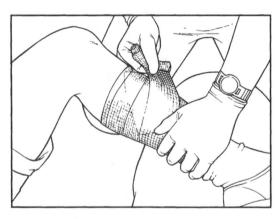

☐ **Apply a pressure bandage**

♦ Using a roller bandage, cover dressing completely, using overlapping turns.

♦ Secure the bandage.

♦ If blood soaks through the bandage, place additional dressings and bandages over the wound.

If bleeding stops...

♦ Determine if further care is needed.

If bleeding does not stop...

♦ Summon more advanced emergency personnel.

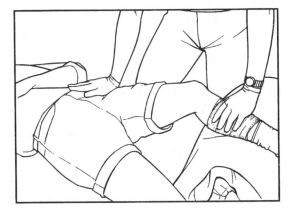

☐ Use a pressure point

◆ Maintain direct pressure and elevation.
◆ Locate femoral artery.
◆ Press the femoral artery against the underlying bone.

Continue to take steps to minimize shock

◆ Maintain direct pressure, elevation, and pressure point.
◆ Position person on back.
◆ Monitor ABCs.
◆ Maintain normal body temperature.
◆ Apply additional dressings and/or bandages as necessary.

PRACTICE SESSION: *Care for a Wound With an Embedded Object*

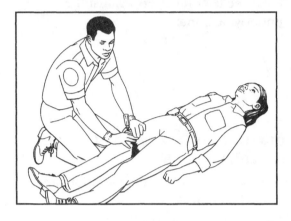

☐ **Apply direct pressure**

   ◆ Avoid moving the body part.
   ◆ Place sterile dressings or clean cloth over the wound, around the object.
   ◆ Press lightly against the wound with your hands.

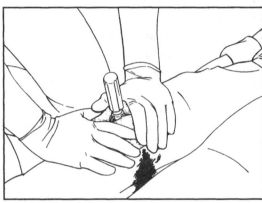

☐ **Support the object**

   ◆ Pack bulky dressings around the object to stabilize it in place.
   ◆ Continue to apply light pressure.

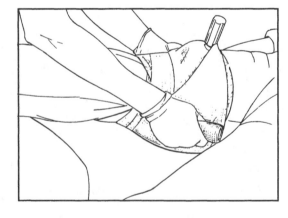

☐ **Apply a pressure bandage**

   ◆ Using a roller bandage, cover the dressings completely, using overlapping turns so that the object is stabilized.

If bleeding stops...

   ◆ Determine if further care is needed.

If bleeding does not stop...

   ◆ Summon more advanced emergency personnel.

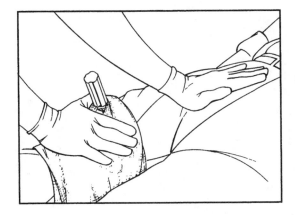

☐ **Use a pressure point**

◆ Maintain direct pressure.
◆ Press the proper pressure point by squeezing the artery against the bone.

Continue to take steps to minimize shock

◆ Maintain direct pressure and pressure point.
◆ Position person on back.
◆ Monitor ABCs.
◆ Maintain normal body temperature.
◆ Apply additional dressings and/or bandages as necessary.

Notes

13

Muscle and Bone Injuries

◆ SUMMARY

The musculoskeletal system has four main structures—bones, muscles, tendons, and ligaments. Sometimes it is difficult to tell whether an injury is a fracture, dislocation, sprain, or strain. Since you cannot be sure which of these conditions a victim might have, always care for the injury as if it were serious. If more advanced medical personnel are on the way, do not move the victim. Control any bleeding first. Take steps to minimize shock, and monitor the ABCs and vital signs. If you are going to transport the victim to a medical facility, be sure to first immobilize the injury before moving the victim.

Any items marked with ** indicate information found only in the Enrichment section of the text.

◆ LEARNING ACTIVITIES

Matching

Match each term with its definition. Write its letter on the line in front of the definition.

Terms

a. Ligament

b. Immobilization

c. Muscle

d. Tendon

e. Splint

Definitions

1. _____ A fibrous band that attaches muscle to bone

2. _____ A tissue that lengthens and shortens to create movement

3. _____ The use of a splint or other method to keep an injured body part from moving

4. _____ A fibrous band that holds bones together at a joint

5. _____ A device used to immobilize a body part

Matching

** Match each term with its definition. Write its letter on the line in front of the definition.

Terms

a. Fracture   e. Thigh

b. Bone   f. Arm

c. Leg   g. Sprain

d. Extremities   h. Strain

Definitions

1. _____ The arms and legs, hands and feet

2. _____ A break or disruption in bone tissue

3. _____ Excessive stretching and tearing of ligaments at a joint

4. _____ The lower extremity between the pelvis and the knee

5. _____ A dense, hard tissue that forms the skeleton

6. _____ Excessive stretching and tearing of muscle tissue

7. _____ The entire lower extremity from the pelvis to the foot

8. _____ The entire upper extremity from the shoulder to the hand

True/False

Circle T if the statement is true; circle F if it is false.

1. T   F   Joints are held together by tough, fibrous connective tissue called tendons.

2. T   F   One of the four types of splints available to the first responder is an improvised splint.

3. T   F   The amount of swelling is, by itself, usually a reliable sign of the severity of a fracture or dislocation.

4. T   F   Tying a victim's fractured leg to the uninjured leg does not effectively splint a fracture.

5. T   F   If a victim cannot bear weight on an ankle or foot, he or she should be evaluated by a physician.

6. T   F   You have splinted a painful, swollen, deformed lower leg. He has no other injuries. It is appropriate to transport him to the hospital yourself rather than calling more advanced medical personnel.

7. T   F   Splinting usually increases the victim's pain.

8. T   F   You might suspect that a victim who heard a pop or a snap at the time of injury has suffered a severe musculoskeletal injury.

9. T   F   Applying ice and elevating the injured part first will usually make it easier to splint a serious musculoskeletal injury.

10. T   F   Muscles are attached to bones by strong, cordlike tissues called ligaments.

11. T   F   Pain when moving a body part is always a sign/symptom of a serious musculoskeletal injury.

**12. T   F   Your care of a closed fracture should include an ice pack over the injury site to help reduce the swelling or pain.

**13. T   F   If more advanced medical personnel have been called to aid a victim of a possible leg fracture who is lying on the ground, the ground can be used as an effective temporary splint until the ambulance arrives.

**14. T   F   Fractures or dislocations of an upper extremity can be effectively immobilized by binding the injured arm to the victim's chest.

15. T F After you splint an extremity, the victim's toes or fingers below the splint should be pale and feel cool.

16. T F You suspect a victim has a fracture of the lower jaw. You should call for assistance from more advanced medical personnel.

17. T F In most sprains, pain, swelling, and any deformity are confined to the joint area.

18. T F In giving care for a sprain, apply heat first and follow by applying cold.

19. T F A sign that leads you to suspect a fractured scapula is deformity of the area.

20. T F To avoid overinflating an air splint, stop inflating it when you can still make a slight dent in the surface of the splint with your thumb.

21. T F Injuries to the elbow can cause permanent disability, since all the nerves and blood vessels to the forearm and hand go through the elbow.

22. T F You find a victim with an injured femur lying with the injured thigh against the ground. You need not move it because the ground provides an effective splint.

23. T F Placing an injured upper arm in a sling and binding it to the chest with cravats is an effective technique for splinting a fracture of the arm.

24. T F To effectively splint an injured ankle and foot, you could use a rigid splint along the back of the leg extending beyond the knee and ankle.

25. T F A fracture of the clavicle is more likely to occur in a child than in an adult.

Short Answer

Read each statement or question and write the correct answer or answers in the space provided.

1. What are the four basic principles of splinting?

2. Explain why applying cold can be helpful in the care of musculoskeletal injuries.

3. What are five common signs and symptoms of most musculoskeletal injuries?

** 6. Describe the three steps for using rigid splints to immobilize a fracture of the lower leg.

4. List the three basic types of mechanisms of injury.

7. List at least four signs and symptoms of a serious extremity injury.

5. What are the five reasons why you would consider immobilizing a serious musculoskeletal injury?

** 8. Why must you check for circulation and sensation below a suspected fracture site before and after splinting?

** 9. Identify the bones of the upper and lower extremities.

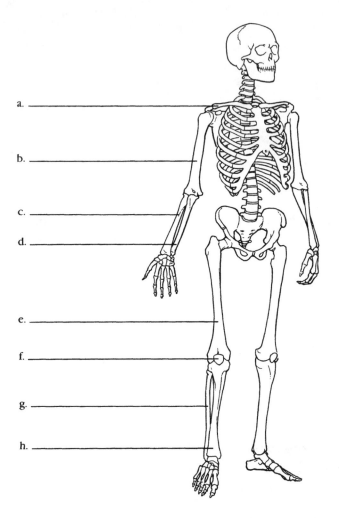

a. _____

b. _____

c. _____

d. _____

e. _____

f. _____

g. _____

h. _____

◆ CASE STUDIES

Read the case studies and answer the questions that follow.

Case 13.1

You are at the scene where a car has struck a pedestrian. The victim is lying on the ground nearby. The scene appears safe. On approaching the victim, you see a bloody wound and significant deformity of the victim's left forearm and thigh.

1. What should be your first step in caring for this victim?

   a. Do a physical examination.

   b. Complete an initial assessment.

   c. Cover the open wound on the forearm.

   d. Check for other less obvious injuries.

2. T F The danger of shock should be addressed by controlling bleeding, elevating the victim's legs, and administering oxygen before completing a physical examination.

3. Since you find no other injuries, you proceed to care for the injuries on the victim's forearm and thigh. Which would be appropriate care for the forearm injury after you have controlled bleeding and covered the wound with a dressing?

   a. Securing the forearm to the victim's body

   b. Splinting the forearm in the position you found it

   c. Gently straightening the forearm before applying a rigid splint and sling

   d. Using an air splint to apply pressure to the wound and straightening the deformity

4. If, after you have splinted the forearm, you note that the fingers of the left hand are bluish in color and feel cool, what should you do?

2. How would you determine whether the injured arm is deformed at the injury site?

   a. Visually compare the injured arm with the victim's uninjured arm.

   b. Apply gentle pressure to see if you can straighten the arm.

   c. Lift the arm gently away from the victim's side and feel for swelling, bumps, or depressions on both sides of the upper arm.

   d. Without moving the arm, gently run your fingers over the exposed surface to determine if there are noticeable bumps or depressions.

3. What three things can you do to help minimize swelling?

4. List three ways you could check for circulation and sensation in the injured arm?

Case 13.2

A young man has been shot in the arm in a hunting accident. He is sitting, holding his arm against his chest. You are a member of the hunting party and the only trained first responder. The victim is conscious and tells you he is in a lot of pain and cannot move his arm. He thinks the bullet broke something. As you assess the injury, you find an entrance and exit wound in the arm above the elbow. There is minimal bleeding.

1. T F The signs and symptoms indicate a good possibility that this victim has a fracture of the humerus.

Case 13.3

A house painter loses his balance and falls from a ladder while painting the second story of a house. You are called to the scene. Bystanders tell you that he landed on his feet and crumpled to the ground. He has not been moved and is lying on his left side. He is conscious, breathing normally, and complaining of pain in both ankles, especially when he tries to move them.

1. T F In this situation, more advanced medical personnel should be called immediately.

2. Given the way the victim landed, what other body parts might you suspect to be injured?

   a. Ribs

   b. Pelvis

   c. Spine

   d. b and c

3. T F As part of your care for this victim, you should apply and maintain in-line stabilization to his head and neck.

4. Describe the care you would provide for this victim's ankle injuries.

**Case 13.4

You are called to the scene of an automobile crash. The driver of one car struck his right forearm on the door handle as the car rolled over. He was wearing his safety belt and has left the car under his own power. He is sitting in the grass at the side of the road, supporting his right forearm, which has a wound with minimal bleeding.

1. Which two bones may be fractured in the forearm?

   a. Humerus and scapula

   b. Tibia and fibula

   c. Radius and ulna

   d. Patella and femur

2. T F To splint this possible fracture, the splint must immobilize both the elbow and wrist.

** 3. Describe how changes in air temperature affect an air splint.

4. T F If you use a rigid splint to immobilize this possible fracture, you should place a roll of gauze in the palm of the victim's hand to keep the palm and fingers in a normal position.

◆ SELF-ASSESSMENT

Circle the letter of the best answer.

1. An effective splint should—

   a. Prevent a closed extremity injury from becoming an open extremity injury.

   b. Lessen pain and increase the victim's comfort.

   c. Reduce the risk of serious internal bleeding.

   d. All of the above.

2. You would suspect a serious musculoskeletal injury if a victim tells you that she—

   a. Has a slight pain in her ankle when she walks.

   b. Has no feeling in her hands.

   c. Has a history of frequent prior dislocations.

   d. Notices that her injured wrist feels warm to the touch.

3. Which of these signs and symptoms indicate that an injury to the foot or ankle needs to be evaluated by a physician?

   a. The foot or ankle is swollen.

   b. The ankle or foot is painful to move.

   c. The victim cannot bear weight on the ankle or foot.

   d. All of the above.

** 4. When treating an elbow with a suspected fracture, you should immobilize the arm—

   a. And then correct any deformity.

   b. In the position in which it was found.

   c. After the arm has been extended.

   d. Only after correcting any deformity.

5. The four types of splints available to the first responder are the soft splint, rigid splint, traction splint, and—

   a. Anatomic splint.

   b. Commercial splint.

   c. Improvised splint.

   d. Flexible splint.

6. Which of the following are part of general care for musculoskeletal injuries?

   a. Ice and gentle exercise

   b. Rest, ice, and elevation

   c. Splints, bandaging, and elevation

   d. Rest and heat packs

7. Which should be part of your emergency care for a victim of a painful, swollen ankle?

   a. An ice pack to decrease swelling and pain

   b. A warm pack to decrease bruising and stiffness

   c. Gentle movement of the joint to retain mobility

   d. A tightly applied elastic bandage to immobilize the joint

8. A child has fallen from a skateboard and landed on an unpadded elbow. What signs/symptoms would you expect to see if the elbow joint is injured?

   a. Inability to move the elbow

   b. Deformity at the elbow

   c. A swollen and/or discolored elbow

   d. All of the above

9. What should you do before splinting this child's arm?

   a. Control any bleeding.

   b. Ask the child to sit up and hold the elbow close to her chest.

   c. Ask the child to carefully attempt to straighten the injured arm.

   d. Apply a warm, moist pack to help reduce the pain.

10. Injuries to the musculoskeletal system are identified and cared for during the—

    a. Initial assessment.

    b. Physical examination.

    c. Scene size-up.

    d. a and b.

**11. When using a rigid splint to treat a painful, swollen, deformed lower leg—

    a. Pad the splint to fit the deformity and secure the splint in place with cravats.

    b. Have a bystander help you straighten the leg before you apply a rigid splint.

    c. Leave the leg unsplinted until the victim can be moved to an ambulance.

    d. Bandage the leg using bulky dressings to immobilize the fractured area.

**12. How can you distinguish a sprain from a strain?

    a. A sprain will usually swell more quickly than a strain.

    b. A sprain is not usually accompanied by deformity, while a strain is often evidenced by deformity.

    c. A sprain usually causes pain and swelling confined to a joint, while the pain and swelling of a strain are usually in areas other than joints.

    d. A strain is usually the result of severe stress or impact, while a sprain is more often the result of a minimal amount of stress or force.

**13. For an injury to be classified as a sprain, which structure must be injured?

    a. Tendon

    b. Cartilage

    c. Ligament

    d. Bone

**14. Which of the following signs indicates a fractured femur?

    a. The leg shortened and foot turned outward

    b. The leg lengthened and foot turned inward

    c. The leg shortened and foot turned inward

    d. The leg lengthened and foot turned outward

**15. How should you immobilize a serious shoulder injury?

    a. Allow the victim to continue to support the arm and immobilize it in that position.

    b. Gently straighten the arm, apply a rigid splint, and secure the arm to the victim's body.

    c. Use pillows, blankets, or other padding to fill any gaps between the arm and the victim's body.

    d. a and c.

**16. Which pattern is most effective for applying a pressure bandage to a shoulder or knee?

    a. Cravat pattern

    b. Figure-eight pattern

    c. Four-tailed pattern

    d. Triangular pattern

**17. Which of the following could you use to splint an injured ankle and foot?

    a. A rigid splint from the lower leg to the foot

    b. A rigid splint along the back of the leg, extending beyond the knee and ankle

    c. An elastic bandage covering from 6 inches above the ankle to the toes

    d. A pillow wrapped around the foot and ankle and secured with 3 cravats

**18. Which is an appropriate way to immobilize a fractured clavicle?

a. Placing the arm on the injured side in a sling

b. Securing the arm on the injured side with a rigid splint reaching from the armpit past the elbow

c. Supporting the arm on the injured side with a sling and binding the arm to the victim's body

d. Having the victim lie on a firm, flat surface and binding the arm on the injured side to the victim's chest

**19. A traction splint is appropriate for—

a. A forearm fracture.

b. A thigh fracture.

c. An ankle fracture.

d. All of the above.

Notes

PRACTICE SESSION: *Applying a Rigid Splint (Forearm)*

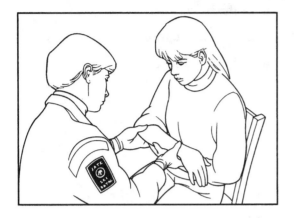

☐ **Support the injured area**

◆ Support above and below injury. If possible, have victim or bystander help you.

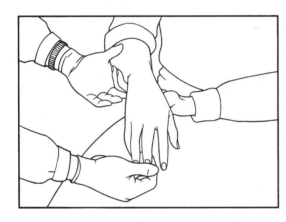

☐ **Check circulation and sensation**

◆ Check for circulation and sensation below the injury.

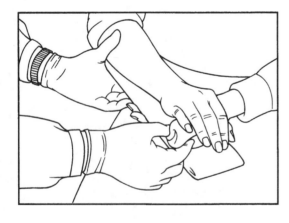

☐ **Position the splint**

◆ Have victim or bystander hold splint in place.
◆ Pad the splint to keep the injured area in a natural position.

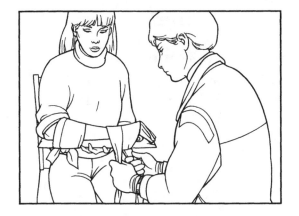

☐ **Secure the splint**

◆ Secure splint above and below injury with cravats or roller bandage.
◆ If cravats are used, leave the injured area uncovered.

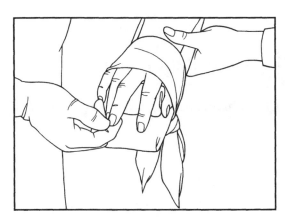

☐ **Recheck circulation and sensation**

◆ Check for circulation and sensation below the injury.
◆ Splint should fit snugly but not so tightly that blood flow is impaired.
◆ If area below the injury is bluish or cool, loosen splint.

PRACTICE SESSION: *Applying a Sling and Binder (Arm)*

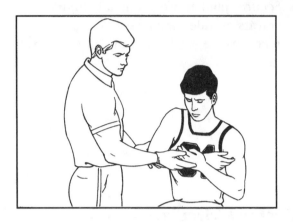

☐ Support the injured area

- ◆ Support above and below injury. If possible, have victim or bystander help you.

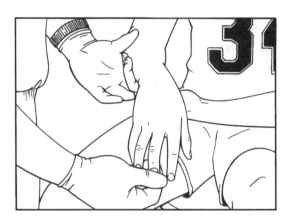

☐ Check circulation and sensation

- ◆ Check hand and fingers for circulation and sensation.

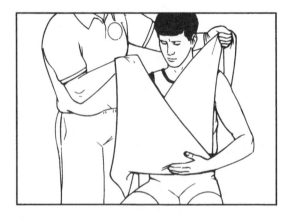

☐ Position the splint

- ◆ Thread one end of bandage under injured arm, across chest, and over uninjured shoulder.
- ◆ Position point of bandage at elbow.
- ◆ Bring other end across chest and over opposite shoulder.

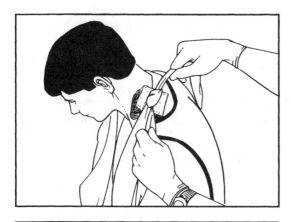

☐ Secure the splint

- ◆ Tie ends of sling at side of neck opposite injury.
- ◆ Placing a pad of gauze under the knot will make it more comfortable.

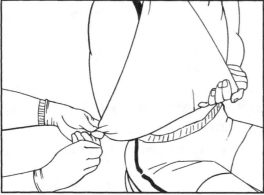

- ◆ Tie or pin points of sling at elbow, if possible.

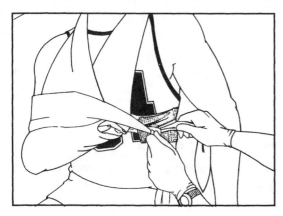

- ◆ Bind arm to chest using a cravat over injured arm.
- ◆ Tie ends of binder on opposite side.
- ◆ Place pad under knot.

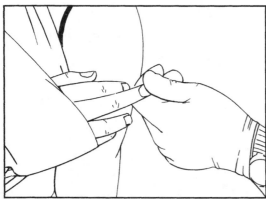

☐ Recheck circulation and sensation

- ◆ Check hand and fingers for circulation and sensation.

PRACTICE SESSION: *Applying an Anatomic Splint (Leg)*

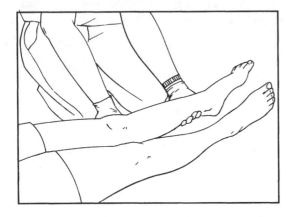

☐ **Support the injured area**

- ◆ Support leg above and below injury.
- ◆ Let the ground support the leg whenever possible.

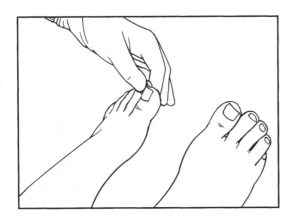

☐ **Check circulation and sensation**

- ◆ Check for circulation and sensation below the injury.

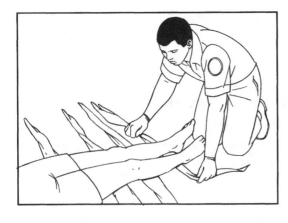

☐ **Position the splint**

- ◆ Thread several cravats above and below the injured area.
- ◆ Do not thread cravat at injury site.

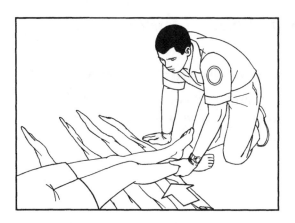

◆ Place uninjured area next to injured area.

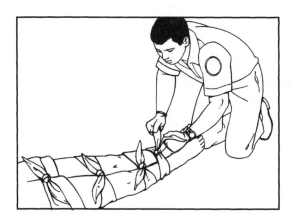

☐ Secure the splint in place

◆ Tie ends of each cravat together, with knots.
◆ Check to see that cravats are snug but not too tight.
◆ If more than 1 finger fits under cravats, tighten cravats.

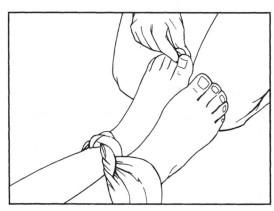

☐ Recheck circulation and sensation

◆ Check for circulation and sensation below the injury.
◆ Splint should fit snugly but not so tightly that blood flow is impaired.
◆ If area below the injury is bluish or cool, loosen splint.

PRACTICE SESSION: *Applying a Soft Splint (Ankle)*

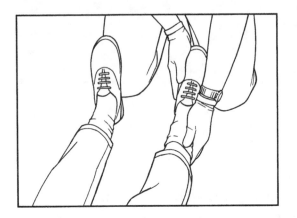

☐ **Support the injured area**

◆ Support above and below injury. If possible, have victim or bystander help you.

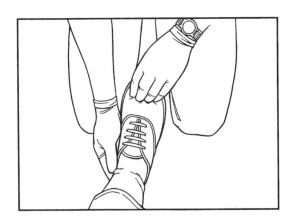

☐ **Check circulation and sensation**

◆ Check for circulation below the injury.

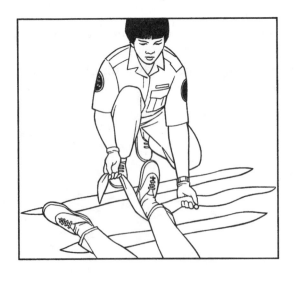

☐ **Position the splint**

◆ Thread several cravats above and below the injury.

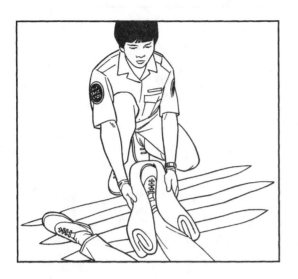

◆ Fold or wrap the splint gently around the injured area.

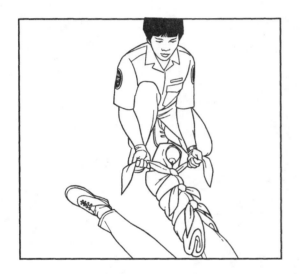

☐ Secure the splint in place

◆ Tie cravats.
◆ For an injury to the ankle, tie cravat around foot, from heel to front of ankle.
◆ If more than 1 finger fits under cravats, tighten cravats.

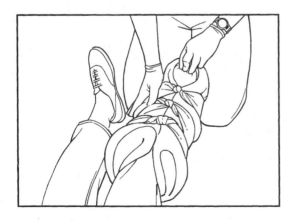

☐ Recheck circulation and sensation

◆ Check for circulation and sensation below the injury.
◆ Splint should fit snugly but not so tightly that blood flow is impaired.
◆ If area below the injury is bluish or cool, loosen splint.

Notes

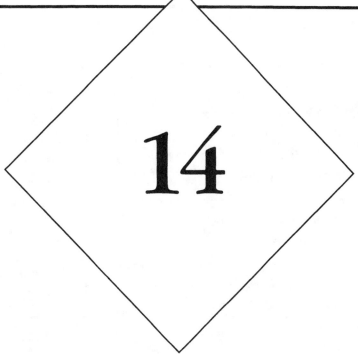

Injuries to the Head, Neck, and Back

◆ SUMMARY

I
n Chapter 14, you learned how to recognize and care for serious head, neck, and
back injuries and specific injuries to the
head and neck. To decide whether an injury
is serious, you must consider its cause. Often
the cause is the best indicator of whether an
injury to the head, neck, or back should be
considered serious. If you have any doubts
about the seriousness of an injury, summon
more advanced medical personnel.

Like injuries elsewhere on the body,
injuries to the head, neck, and back often
involve both soft tissues and bone. Control
bleeding as necessary, usually with direct
pressure on the wound. With scalp injuries,
be careful not to apply pressure to a possible
skull fracture. With eye injuries, remember
not to apply pressure on the eyeball.

If you suspect that the victim may have a
serious head, neck, or back injury, minimize
movement of the injured area when providing care. Minimizing movement is best
accomplished by using in-line stabilization.
Administer oxygen if it is available and you
are trained to do so. Apply a cervical collar
and secure the victim to a backboard if you
must move the victim.

Any items marked with ** indicate information found only in the Enrichment section of the text.

◆ LEARNING ACTIVITIES

Matching

Match each term with its definition. Write its letter on the line in front of the definition.

Terms

a. Spinal column

b. Concussion

c. Cervical collar

d. Vertebrae

e. Spinal cord

f. In-line stabilization

g. Disks

Definitions

1. _____ Cushions of cartilage separating vertebrae

2. _____ A series of bones extending from the base of the skull to the tip of the tailbone

3. _____ A rigid device positioned around the neck to limit movement of the head and neck

4. _____ A temporary impairment of brain function

5. _____ Small irregular bones with circular openings in the center; form the backbone

6. _____ A technique used to minimize movement of a victim's head and neck

7. _____ Carries sensory and motor impulses between the brain and other areas of the body

True/False

Circle T if the statement is true; circle F if it is false.

1. T F In caring for a penetrating wound of the eye, you should close and cover the victim's uninjured eye.

2. T F You should expect to feel some resistance when bringing the head of a victim who may have a back injury in line with the body. You should continue gently moving the head until it is in the anatomically normal position.

3. T F The most common cause of head, neck, and back injuries is diving into shallow water.

4. T F A knocked-out tooth should be preserved in milk, or water if milk is not available, and transported with the victim for possible replantation.

5. T F A person has a gunshot wound in the abdomen. You should care for the victim as a possible spinal injury victim.

6. T F Victims of severe head, neck, or back injuries are unlikely to suffer from shock.

** 7. T F Inspecting work and recreational equipment periodically is a safety practice that can help prevent injuries to the head, neck, and back.

** 8. T F If a backboard or an adequate number of trained personnel are not available for immobilizing a suspected head, neck, and back injury victim, a first responder should support the victim in the position in which he or she is found until more advanced medical personnel arrive.

9. T F A person is found unconscious with no wounds or bleeding from the head. The victim is unlikely to have a serious head injury.

10. T F Nausea and vomiting are among the signs and symptoms of head, neck, and/or back injuries.

11. T F To control bleeding from a wound on the scalp, you should immediately apply firm direct pressure over the wound with a clean dressing.

12. T F You should not move the victim's head in-line with the body if the victim complains of pain or pressure in the neck when you begin to align the head with the body.

13. T F In most cases, the proper position for a victim of a nosebleed is sitting with the head tilted back.

14. T F You should not remove a foreign object from a victim's ear canal even if the object can be easily dislodged.

15. T F A victim suspected of having a concussion does not need to be seen by advanced medical personnel.

16. T F It is important to monitor the vital signs of a victim with a head, neck, and back injury because the chest nerves and muscles can become paralyzed and breathing can stop.

Short Answer

Read each statement or question and write the correct answer or answers in the space provided.

1. What are the three circumstances in which you would **not** move the head of a spinal injury victim in line with the body?

2. What are three situations in which you should summon more advanced medical personnel to deal with a nosebleed?

3. List at least five situations that would lead you to consider the possibility of serious head, neck, and/or back injuries.

4. What are the six steps of care to be performed for an eye injury involving an embedded object?

5. List at least seven signs and symptoms that could indicate a victim has suffered a head, neck, and/or back injury.

** 6. Describe the five steps for immobilizing a victim with a head, neck, and/or back injury if at least two first responders are present and you have a backboard.

** 7. List at least four safety practices that can help prevent head, neck, and back injuries.

◆ CASE STUDIES

Read the case studies and answer the questions that follow.

Case 14.1

A young man has fallen from the roof of his two-story house to the ground. You are called to the scene. You find the man unconscious but breathing normally. He has an abrasion on his forehead and blood trickling from his mouth. You see no other signs of injury.

1. What would you do next in caring for this victim?

   a. Monitor vital signs.

   b. Establish an open airway.

   c. Minimize movement of the head and spine.

   d. Control the bleeding from his forehead.

2. Explain why a closed head injury suffered by this victim may become a life-threatening problem.

3. The victim's head is turned to the left side as he lies on his back. Under which of the following circumstances would you not move his head in line with his body as part of your emergency care?

   a. You see drainage of clear fluid and blood from his left ear.

   b. His head is severely angled to one side.

   c. A second rescuer arrives, enabling you to care for the victim without moving his head.

   d. You find a medical identification tag that indicates the victim has a history of seizures.

4. You have applied in-line stabilization, moving the victim's head in line with his body. As you tell a bystander to call for advanced medical help, the victim begins to vomit. Which of the following should you do?

a. Turn the victim's head to the side and sweep out the vomit with your fingers.

b. Keep the victim's head in line with the body and have the bystander sweep out the vomit with his or her fingers.

c. Turn the victim's head to the side and maintain in-line stabilization while the vomit drains from his mouth.

d. Ask the bystander to assist in log-rolling the victim's body to one side while you maintain in-line stabilization.

** 5. T F In securing this victim's head to a backboard, rolled towels can be used to restrict the victim's head from moving from side to side.

Case 14.2

A young woman swerved her car to avoid striking a dog. Her car rolled over and off the roadway. She struck her cheek and jaw on the side window, which shattered during the rollover. She is bleeding from a puncture wound that goes completely through the left cheek. Two of her teeth are missing in the area of the wound. She is conscious, has gotten out of the car, and is holding her hand against her cheek. She sits down while you examine her.

1. How should you control the bleeding from this victim's cheek?

a. Apply direct pressure to the outside of the cheek with a dressing and have the victim hold it in place.

b. Place several folded dressings inside her mouth against the cheek and have the victim hold them in place.

c. Place dressings on both the outside and inside of the cheek and apply direct pressure with the victim's hand or a pressure bandage.

d. Apply pressure to the facial artery pressure point and place several dressings inside the mouth against the cheek.

2. Describe how you could control bleeding from the gums in the area from which her two teeth were dislodged.

3. T F The best method for preserving the dislodged teeth for replantation is to place them in the victim's mouth.

4. It is important that a dislodged tooth be replanted in its socket within—

a. Thirty minutes after the injury.

b. One hour after the injury.

c. One and one-half hours after the injury.

d. Two hours after the injury.

◆ SELF-ASSESSMENT

Circle the letter of the best answer.

1. Which of the following may indicate a head, neck, or back injury?

   a. Tingling in the extremities

   b. Partial or complete loss of movement of any body part

   c. Loss of balance

   d. All of the above

2. Nearly half of all head, neck, and back injuries are the result of—

   a. Sport's accidents.

   b. Motor vehicle collisions.

   c. Falls from heights.

   d. Assaults and attacks.

3. In which of the following situations should you consider the possibility of a serious head, neck, and/or back injury?

   a. An adult who fell from a height of 4 feet

   b. A construction worker whose safety cap was cracked when he was struck by a dropped hammer

   c. A conscious victim of a motor vehicle crash who was not wearing a seat belt

   d. b and c

4. An appropriate bandage for controlling bleeding from the neck is—

   a. A pressure bandage so it does not restrict blood flow.

   b. A bulky bandage taped directly over the wound.

   c. A loosely wrapped bandage fully encircling the neck.

   d. An encircling bandage that applies pressure to the carotid arteries.

5. A small piece of glass has become embedded in a victim's eye. The victim has no other injuries or problems. What would you do first in caring for this victim?

   a. Place a sterile dressing around the object and control bleeding surrounding the eye.

   b. Stabilize the object with bulky dressings and a paper cup to secure it in place.

   c. Place the victim on the back, reassuring him or her and cautioning not to move the eyes.

   d. Cover the uninjured eye to prevent blinking or other eye movement that might increase eye damage.

6. How should you attempt to control bleeding from a scalp wound in which the skull appears depressed?

   a. Direct pressure on the wound

   b. Pressure on the temporal point

   c. Pressure on the area around the wound

   d. A sterile dressing only; no pressure

** 7 To help prevent head, neck, and back injuries, you should—

   a. Avoid inappropriate use of drugs.

   b. Inspect mechanical equipment before use.

   c. Follow the rules in sports activities.

   d. All of the above.

** 8 In securing a victim to a backboard, use straps or cravats to secure the victim's—

   a. Chest and thighs.

   b. Chest, hips, thighs, and legs.

   c. Hips, thighs, and legs.

   d. Hips and legs.

** 9. A victim is wearing a full face motor-cycle helmet. In which of the following circumstances would you remove the helmet?

   a. A bystander states that it should be removed.

   b. When you are unable to assess or care for airway and breathing problems.

   c. It interferes with efforts to stabilize the head.

   d. b and c.

Notes

PRACTICE SESSION: *Controlling Bleeding for an Open Head Wound*

Using the steps below, practice bandaging the scalp, cheek, and neck. Refer to Chapter 14 of your textbook for assistance.

☐ **Apply direct pressure**

◆ Place sterile dressing or clean cloth over wound and press gently against wound with your hand.

◆ Do not put direct pressure on wound if you feel depression, spongy area, or bone fragments.

◆ Press gently on area around wound.

☐ **Elevate the body part**

◆ Elevate the head and shoulders unless you suspect an injury to the spine.

☐ **Apply a pressure bandage**

◆ Using a roller bandage, cover dressing completely, using overlapping turns.

◆ Tie or tape bandage in place.

◆ If blood soaks through bandage, place additional dressings and bandages over wound.

If bleeding stops...

◆ Determine if further care is needed.

If bleeding does not stop...

◆ Summon more advanced emergency personnel.

PRACTICE SESSION: *Bandaging an Eye With an Embedded Object*

☐ **Position the victim**
   ◆ Position victim on back.

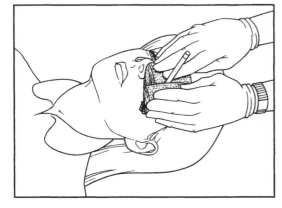

☐ **Support the object**
   ◆ Place sterile dressings around object.
   ◆ Place a bulky dressing around the object to help support it.

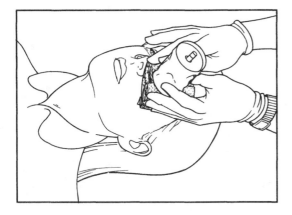

☐ ◆ If available, place a paper cup over object to stabilize it.

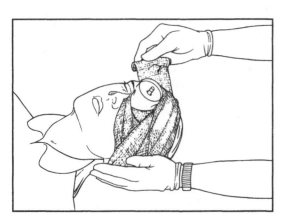

☐ **Apply a bandage**
   ◆ Using a roller bandage, cover dressings completely, using overlapping turns until object is stabilized.

PRACTICE SESSION: *Immobilizing a Head, Neck, or Back Injury*

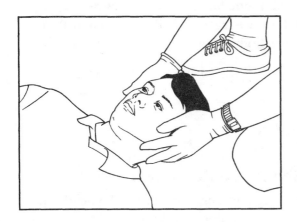

☐ **Apply in-line stabilization**
- ◆ Place your hands on both sides of victim's head.
- ◆ Gently position head in line with body, if necessary.
- ◆ Support head in that position.

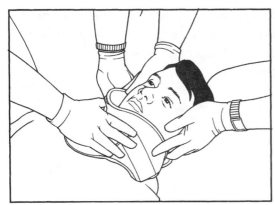

☐ **Apply cervical collar**
- ◆ One rescuer maintains in-line stabilization.
- ◆ Second rescuer applies appropriately sized cervical collar.

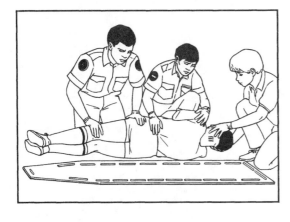

☐ **Log-roll victim onto backboard**
- ◆ One rescuer maintains in-line stabilization of head.
- ◆ Additional rescuers support victim's shoulders, hips, and legs.
- ◆ Roll victim in unison, keeping head and spine in alignment until victim is resting on side.
- ◆ Position backboard.
- ◆ Log-roll the victim onto backboard.

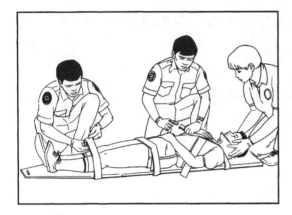

☐ **Secure victim's body**

- ◆ Secure victim's chest.
- ◆ Secure victim's arms, hips, thighs, and legs with remaining straps or cravats.
- ◆ If necessary, secure the hands in front of the body.

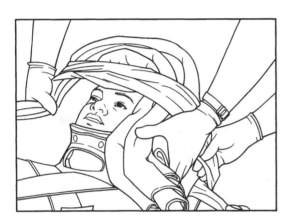

☐ **Secure victim's head**

- ◆ Place padding beneath head if head is not resting in line with body.
- ◆ If commercial head immobilizer is not available, place folded or rolled blanket around head and neck.
- ◆ Secure forehead.

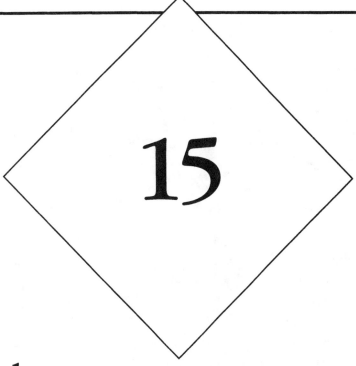

Medical and Behavioral Emergencies

◆ SUMMARY

Medical emergencies can strike anyone at any time. The signs and symptoms of different emergencies are similar, such as changes in the level of consciousness, confusion, weakness, and ill appearance. Recognizing the general signs and symptoms of medical emergencies will indicate the initial care you should provide. Usually, you will not know the cause of the illness. Altered mental status, diabetic emergencies, seizures, and heat- and cold-related emergencies each have an individual, specific cause. Fortunately, you can provide proper care without knowing the cause. Following the general guidelines of care for any emergency will help prevent the condition from becoming worse. When providing care for sudden illnesses, you should—

- Do no further harm.
- Conduct an initial assessment, physical exam, and SAMPLE history.
- Summon more advanced medical personnel.
- Help the victim rest comfortably.
- Keep the victim from getting chilled or overheated.
- Administer oxygen if it is available and you are trained to do so.

When responding to a victim with a possible behavioral emergency, begin by assessing the scene for dangers. Do not assess the victim until law enforcement personnel have secured the scene. Approach the victim cautiously, without making any rapid movements. Attempt to determine the victim's problem, gain consent, and provide any care. If the victim's behavior becomes threatening or violent, attempt to calm the victim. If attempts to calm the victim do not work, you may have to leave the scene. In some situations, reasonable force may be needed to restrain the victim for safe transport to a receiving facility. Document the situation carefully to avoid legal problems in the future.

◆ OUTLINE

Any items marked with ** indicate information found only in the Enrichment section of the text.

◆ LEARNING ACTIVITIES

Matching

Match each term with its definition. Write its letter on the line in front of the definition.

Terms

a. Epilepsy

b. Fainting

c. Seizure

d. Frostbite

e. Hypothermia

Definitions

1. _____ General body cooling

2. _____ A chronic condition characterized by seizures that vary in type and duration

3. _____ Localized cold exposure resulting in body tissue freezing

4. _____ A partial or complete loss of consciousness resulting from a temporary reduction of blood flow to the brain

5. _____ A disorder of the brain's electrical activity, marked by loss of consciousness and often by uncontrollable muscle activity

**Matching

Match each term with its definition. Write its letter on the line in front of the definition

Terms

a. Hypoglycemia

b. Diabetic ketoacidosis

c. Insulin

d. Stroke

e. Hypertension

Definitions

1. _____ A life-threatening emergency in which the body needs insulin

2. _____ A condition in which the body lacks blood sugar

3. _____ A hormone that enables the body to use sugar for energy

4. _____ High blood pressure

5. _____ A disruption of blood to a part of the brain, causing permanent damage

True/False

Circle T if the statement is true; circle F if it is false.

1.   T   F   A person about to faint will frequently resemble a person who is going into shock.

2.   T   F   Febrile (heat-induced) seizures are most common in the elderly.

3.   T   F   Rubbing alcohol should be used to rapidly cool a victim of heat-related illness.

4.   T   F   Severe hypothermia is characterized by severe shivering.

5.   T   F   To help avoid heat-related illness, you should wear dark-colored cotton clothing when working in the heat.

6.   T   F   In advanced stages of heat-related illness, the victim's body loses the ability to remove heat, and its temperature rises to dangerous levels.

7.   T   F   You should place an object between the victim's teeth when caring for a victim having a seizure.

8.   T   F   To care for a fainting victim, elevate the victim's legs.

9.   T   F   An aura is an unusual sensation or feeling that frequently precedes a seizure.

10.   T   F   You do not necessarily need to summon more advanced medical personnel immediately if the victim is known to have periodic seizures, even if the victim has repeated seizures.

11.   T   F   To choose the right emergency care for a victim of a sudden illness, you must be able to identify the illness that is causing the signs and symptoms you note.

12.   T   F   A victim experiencing the early stage of heat-related illness frequently has dry, pale skin, elevated body temperature, and a slow pulse.

13.   T   F   When caring for frostbite, immerse the affected area in hot water for 20–30 minutes.

14.   T   F   Blood vessels near the surface of the victim's skin play a role in the movement of excess heat out of the body.

15. T F Rapid rewarming of a hypothermia victim may trigger dangerous disturbances in the victim's heart rhythm.

16. T F Your personal safety should be a foremost concern when encountering a victim with a behavioral emergency.

17. T F You should speak forcefully and assume an authoritative position when dealing with a victim with a behavioral emergency.

18. T F You should attempt to humor or "play along" with the delusions of a victim with a behavioral emergency.

**19. T F A victim who is suffering from a stroke should be given something to drink to prevent dehydration.

**20. T F Although hyperglycemia and hypoglycemia are different conditions, their major signs and symptoms are similar.

Short Answer

Read each statement or question and write the correct answer or answers in the space provided.

1. List at least four signs and symptoms of medical emergencies.

2. List at least five general guidelines for the assessment and care of medical emergencies.

3. List at least five circumstances in which you would summon more advanced medical personnel to treat a victim of a seizure.

4. Should a first responder try to diagnose the exact cause of an injury or illness? Why or why not?

5. List at least five causes of altered mental status.

◆ CASE STUDIES

Read the case studies and answer the questions that follow.

Case 15.1

A 72-year-old woman becomes confused and wanders out of her house in her bare feet. The outside temperature is 20 degrees Fahrenheit and there is snow on the ground. When you find her, she is conscious, having difficulty speaking, and does not remember what happened. She says that her feet are numb. They look white and waxy.

1. Which of the following conditions is responsible for the condition of her feet?

   a. Stroke

   b. Hypothermia

   c. Altered mental status

   d. Frostbite

2. List the signs and symptoms of frostbite you find in the scenario.

3. After you remove her from the snow, how would you care for this victim's feet?

   a. Rub the feet vigorously to restore circulation.

   b. Wrap the feet snugly in a moist, warm dressing.

   c. Cover the feet with dry dressings and bandage loosely.

   d. Break any blisters that appear and cleanse the foot with soap and water.

4. T F This victim should be seen by more advanced medical personnel as soon as possible.

Case 15.2

It is well into double overtime in a championship basketball game between two long-time rival high schools. The gymnasium is hot. One of the players appears confused and looks ill. The trainer notes that she is breathing rapidly, her pulse is rapid and weak, and her skin is sweaty. The player seems confused about the day and location of the game. The trainer also knows that the player is a diabetic.

1. Which of the following conditions is this player most likely experiencing?

   a. Hypoglycemia

   b. Hyperglycemia

   c. Heat-related illness

   d. a and c

2. What additional information might better help you to decide the victim's condition?

3. What care should be provided to this victim?

Case 15.3

You are giving a presentation to a group of school students when one of the male students cries out and slips from his seat to the floor. You see his muscles tighten and his teeth clench. As you get to his side, he begins to shake uncontrollably and strikes his arm against the leg of his chair.

1. What type of medical emergency is this person probably experiencing?

   a. Transient ischemic attack

   b. Fainting

   c. Seizure

   d. Stroke

2. Which of the following is part of your care for this victim?

   a. Placing something between the victim's teeth

   b. Monitoring and maintaining the victim's airway

   c. Restraining the victim's movements

   d. a and b

3. To protect the victim from injury, you would do all of the following except—

   a. Move away nearby objects that could cause injury.

   b. Hold his arms still.

   c. Position him on his side, if possible, to protect his airway.

   d. Place a thin cushion or folded piece of clothing under his head.

4. Advanced medical personnel should be called if—

   a. He has repeated seizures.

   b. He fails to regain consciousness.

   c. You are uncertain what caused the seizure.

   d. All of the above.

◆ SELF-ASSESSMENT

Circle the letter of the best answer.

1. Steps for preventing both heat- and cold-related illnesses include—

   a. Avoiding being outdoors in the hottest or coldest parts of the day.

   b. Wearing dark colored clothing when in the sun.

   c. Drinking adequate fluids.

   d. a and c.

2. While you are providing emergency care to a victim of a heat-related illness, which of the following signs indicates that you should immediately call more advanced medical personnel?

   a. The victim loses consciousness.

   b. The victim refuses water or vomits.

   c. The victim begins to sweat profusely.

   d. a and b.

3. Which of the following should you do to care for a victim of hypothermia?

   a. Immerse the victim in warm water.

   b. Gradually rewarm the victim.

   c. Rub the victim's arms and legs briskly.

   d. All of the above.

4. Signs of heat-related illness include—

   a. Headache and nausea.

   b. Cool, moist, pale or ashen skin.

   c. Dizziness and weakness.

   d. All of the above.

5. If a victim of a suspected heat-related illness begins to lose consciousness, you should—

   a. Cool the body using wet sheets or towels or cold packs.

   b. Cool the body by applying rubbing alcohol.

   c. Summon more advanced medical personnel.

   d. a and c.

6. Which of the following is a reason to summon more advanced medical assistance during or after a seizure?

   a. The victim regains consciousness.

   b. You are certain about what caused the seizure.

   c. The seizure takes place in water.

   d. The victim is known to have epilepsy.

7. Your emergency care for a victim of fainting should include—

   a. Loosening restrictive clothing.

   b. Sponging the victim's face with a wet towel.

   c. Placing the victim in a semi-sitting position.

   d. Giving a conscious victim small sips of water.

8. Which of the following would be considered to indicate a medical emergency?

   a. Nausea and vomiting

   b. Change in level of consciousness

   c. Changes in pulse and breathing rate

   d. All of the above

** 9. What is the best position in which to place a stroke victim who is drooling or having difficulty swallowing?

   a. Semi-sitting, head raised

   b. Lying on one side

   c. Lying flat on the back

   d. Lying on the back, legs elevated

**10. Which of the following should be included in your emergency care for a diabetic who has signs and symptoms of a diabetic emergency?

   a. Administering oxygen

   b. Injecting insulin into him or her

   c. Giving the person a nondiet cola or fruit juice to drink

   d. a and c

Notes

Notes

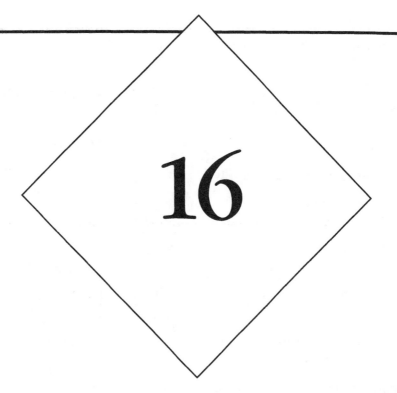

Poisoning

◆ **SUMMARY**

Poisonings can occur in four ways: ingestion, inhalation, absorption, and injection. Substance abuse and misuse are types of poisoning that can occur in any of these ways. Substance abuse and misuse can produce a variety of signs and symptoms, most of which are common to other types of poisoning. You do not need to be able to determine the cause of a poisoning to provide appropriate initial care. If you see any of the signs and symptoms of sudden illness, follow the basic guidelines for care for any medical emergency. For suspected poisonings, contact your local or regional poison control center (PCC) or summon more advanced medical personnel. Beyond following the general guidelines for giving care for a suspected poisoning, medical professionals may advise you to provide some specific care, such as neutralizing the poison with activated charcoal.

Six major categories of substances, when abused or misused, can produce a variety of signs and symptoms, some of which are indistinguishable from those of other medical emergencies. Remember, you do not have to know specific condition to provide care. If you suspect that the victim's condition is caused by substance misuse or abuse, provide care for a poisoning emergency.

◆ **LEARNING ACTIVITIES**

Matching

Match each term with its definition. Write its letter on the line in front of the definition.

Terms

a. Activated charcoal

b. Poison

c. Syrup of ipecac

d. Designer drug

e. Drug

f. Hallucinogen

g. Stimulant

h. Anaphylaxis

i. Overdose

j. Substance abuse

k. Substance misuse

Definitions

1. _____ The use of a substance for unintended purposes, or for appropriate purposes but in improper amounts or doses

2. _____ A substance that absorbs ingested poison

3. _____ A substance that affects mood and thought, alters perceptions of time and space, and produces delusions

4. _____ A medical substance that is chemically modified for street use

5. _____ Deliberate, persistent, excessive use of a substance without regard to health concerns

6. _____ A substance that affects the central nervous system to speed up physical and mental activity

7. _____ A substance used to induce vomiting in poisoning cases

8. _____ A situation in which a person takes enough of a substance that it has poisonous or fatal effects

9. _____ A substance that causes injury or death when introduced into the body

10. _____ A severe allergic reaction; a form of shock

11. _____ Any substance other than food intended to affect the functions of the body

True/False

Circle T if the statement is true; circle F if it is false.

1. T F You should apply an ice or cold pack to the site of a snakebite as soon as possible to slow the absorption of the venom.

2. T F The immediate care for emergencies caused by substance abuse follows the same general principles as the care for any poisoning.

3. T F The four ways poisons enter the body are ingestion, injection, inhalation, and insufflation.

4. T F To prevent poisonings, medications and other potentially dangerous products should be kept in their original containers.

5. T F As a first responder to a possible poisoning, your responsibilities include evaluating the scene and the condition of the victim and getting any available information from bystanders.

6. T F The physical effects you would notice in a person who had ingested a hallucinogenic drug would be similar to those produced by a depressant.

7. T F If you suspect that a conscious victim has been exposed to a poison you should contact 9-1-1 or other local emergency number.

8. T F In cases of exposure to a wet chemical, flush the area with running water.

9. T F Anaphylaxis develops slowly and, in an emergency situation, is often overshadowed by more obvious medical problems.

10. T F You suspect a poisoning. You should try to discover whether the victim has a history of drug misuse or abuse. This information is needed to help you decide the initial care you will provide.

11. T F Once a tick has been removed from the skin, you should wash the area of the bite with soap and water and coat it with an antiseptic ointment.

12. T F If the victim of a poisoning vomits, you should save some of the vomitus as a clue to the nature of the poison.

13. T F At a poisoning scene, you should try to discover the type and amount of poison taken, and how long ago it was taken.

14. T F Caffeine and nicotine are both categorized as stimulants.

15. T F You should try to calm a victim of drug abuse who becomes violent or threatening.

16. T F A victim who appears to be very excited, restless, and talkative might be abusing stimulants.

17. T F If dry chemicals contact the skin, you should flush the affected area continuously with large amounts of running water or brush the chemical off the skin with a gloved hand.

18. T F In caring for a victim of an inhaled poison, you should immediately remove the person from the source of the poison without first surveying the scene.

19. T F Applying warm, moist packs to insect stings will help reduce pain and swelling.

20. T F The care for jellyfish stings is to rub the area with sand and soak it in salt water.

Short Answer

Read each statement or question and write the correct answer or answers in the space provided.

1. List four things you should not do for a victim of snakebite.

2. What are three questions to ask regarding a suspected poisoning?

3. List the four ways in which a poison can enter the body.

4. List at least five signs and symptoms of anaphylaxis.

5. What is the usual dose of activated charcoal for children?

◆ CASE STUDIES

Read the case studies and answer the questions that follow.

Case 16.1

In a softball tournament, one of the players retrieves a foul ball and play continues. About 15 minutes later, the girl complains of tightness in her throat. She is perspiring heavily. As you examine her, you note hives on her body.

1. Which of the following would likely be the cause of this girl's problem?

    a. Black widow spider

    b. Tick

    c. Scorpion

    d. Bee

2. Which of these is least likely to have caused her problem, and why?

3. As you care for this girl, her condition worsens. She begins to have serious difficulty breathing and you hear wheezing. What condition do you suspect is developing?

    a. Rabies

    b. Tetanus

    c. Anaphylaxis

    d. Lyme disease

4. T F Part of your treatment for this victim should be to administer oxygen and summon more advanced medical personnel.

5. Which of the following medications might this girl carry or her parents have available that could ease her symptoms?

    a. Nitroglycerine

    b. Epinephrine

    c. Insulin

    d. Codeine

Case 16.2

You are called late one evening to respond to a man lying in the doorway of a building. You find a middle-age man lying on the sidewalk. He is thin, flushed, and sweating profusely. He has recently vomited. He tries to push you away when you first attempt to touch him and mutters something about getting "the rattlesnakes" away from him. When you try to speak with him or ask him questions, he simply moans or grunts. After a few moments, he becomes unresponsive. His pulse rate is 100 and his respiration rate is 28 and breaths are shallow.

1. T F Proper emergency care for this victim depends on your ability to determine whether this is a case of substance abuse or a medical condition not related to substance use.

2. T F This victim's signs and symptoms are consistent with use of hallucinogen drugs.

3. Which of the following are included in the general principles you will use in treating this victim?

    a. Summon more advanced medical personnel.

    b. Try to keep the victim calm by minimizing movement.

    c. Attempt to find bystanders who are familiar with the victim.

    d. All of the above.

4. What should you do if the victim becomes violent or threatening?

   a. Try to physically restrain him.

   b. Ignore him and continue to provide care.

   c. Withdraw to a safe distance and wait for more advanced personnel.

   d. Ask bystanders to help you.

◆ SELF-ASSESSMENT

Circle the letter of the best answer.

1. Which signs and symptoms are you likely to find in a victim of anaphylaxis?

   a. Hives, rash, and itching

   b. Nausea and vomiting

   c. Coughing and wheezing

   d. All of the above

2. Which of the following is the typical first sign of an infection resulting from a deer tick bite?

   a. A rash

   b. Dry flaky patches

   c. Small blisters

   d. Numerous red, swollen areas

3. Which of the following signs and symptoms would help you distinguish a victim of poisoning from a victim of another medical emergency?

   a. Nausea, vomiting, and abdominal pain

   b. Breathing difficulty and faintness

   c. Burns around the lips and tongue

   d. Seizures and loss of consciousness

4. Which of the following questions should you ask about a suspected poisoning to help you provide emergency care?

   a. How much was taken?

   b. When was the poison taken?

   c. Does the victim have a history of drug use/abuse?

   d. a and b.

5. Which of the following can be the source of an injected poison?

   a. A house fly

   b. An aspirin

   c. A bathroom cleaner

   d. A wasp

6. Which signs and symptoms are you likely to find in a person who has taken an overdose of depressants?

   a. Slurred speech, drowsiness, and confusion

   b. Paranoia, rapid pulse, and pinpoint pupils

   c. Sweating, chills, and rapid pulse

   d. Euphoria, dry skin, and flushed face

7. Which of the following is likely to be helpful as a general guideline to help prevent poisonings?

   a. Keep all medications within reach.

   b. Place all prescription medication in marked bottles.

   c. Keep products in their original containers with their original labels in place.

   d. Do not dispose of outdated products.

8. Where would you be most likely to find a Poison Control Center?

    a. In the emergency department of a large hospital

    b. In a city or county health department

    c. In a large police or fire department

    d. All of the above

9. Which of the following might be used in caring for a poisoning victim?

    a. Activated charcoal

    b. Paregoric

    c. Syrup of ipecac

    d. a and c

10. Which of the following are major categories of commonly abused or misused substances?

    a. Medications, alcohol, and cocaine

    b. Stimulants, hallucinogens, and depressants

    c. Inhalants, amphetamines, and narcotics

    d. Alcohol, cocaine, and heroin

Notes

Notes

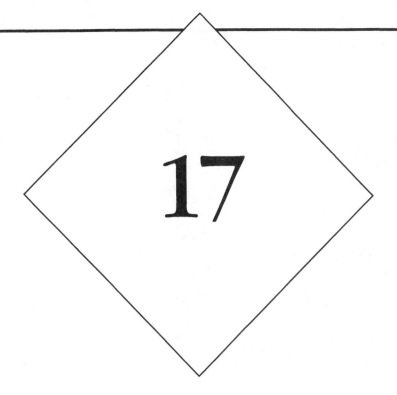

Childbirth

◆ SUMMARY

I deally, childbirth should occur in a controlled environment under the guidance of healthcare professionals trained in delivery. In this situation, the necessary medical care is immediately available for mother and baby should any problem arise. However, unexpected deliveries do occur outside of the controlled environment and may require your assistance. By understanding the four stages of labor and knowing how to prepare the expectant mother for delivery, assist in the delivery, and provide proper care for the mother and baby, you will be able to successfully assist in bringing a new child into the world.

◆ OUTLINE

Any items marked with ** indicate information found only in the Enrichment section of the text.

◆ LEARNING ACTIVITIES

Matching

Match each term with its definition. Write its letter on the line in front of the definition.

Terms

a. Amniotic sac   f. Crowning

b. Birth canal   g. Labor

c. Placenta   h. Cervix

d. Umbilical cord   i. Contraction

e. Bloody show   j. Uterus

Definitions

1. _____ A pear-shaped organ in a woman's pelvis in which a fertilized egg develops into a baby

2. _____ A rhythmic tightening of certain muscles during delivery

3. _____ The process which begins with contractions of the uterus and ends with the stabilization and recovery of the mother

4. _____ An organ attached to the uterus that supplies nutrients to the fetus

5. _____ The appearance of the baby's head at the vaginal opening

6. _____ The upper part of the birth canal

7. _____ A fluid-filled structure that protects the developing fetus

8. _____ A flexible structure that attaches the placenta to the fetus; carries blood, nutrients, and waste

9. _____ Pink or light red thick discharge from the vagina that occurs during labor

10. _____ The passageway from the uterus to the vaginal opening through which the baby passes during birth

**Matching

Match each term with its definition. Write its letter on the line in front of the definition.

Terms

a. Breech birth

b. Prolapsed cord

c. Miscarriage

Definitions

1. _____ A complication of childbirth in which a loop of the umbilical cord slips through the vaginal opening prior to delivery of the baby

2. _____ Delivery of a baby's feet or buttocks at the vaginal opening before the head

3. _____ A spontaneous end to pregnancy before the twentieth week

True/False

Circle T if the statement is true; circle F if it is false.

1. T F Taking a childbirth class can help you become more competent in techniques to help expectant mothers relax.

2. T F Crowning is the point in a delivery at which the baby's head is visible at the opening of the vagina.

3. T F One purpose of your assistance in the birth of a baby is to help guide the baby from the vaginal opening.

4. T F After delivery, it is important to get the mother up and walking as soon as possible.

5. T F A bulb syringe is helpful for suctioning secretions from the newborn's nose and mouth.

6. T F To time contractions, you start timing at the end of one contraction until the beginning of the next one.

7. T F One of the factors that you need to determine about the mother's condition when she is in labor is whether the amniotic sac has ruptured.

8. T F When caring for a newborn, one of your critical responsibilities is to maintain a clear airway.

9. T F Shocklike signs and symptoms in the mother are rare in childbirth situations immediately after giving birth.

10. T F Stage four of the labor process is when the placenta separates from the uterine wall and exits from the birth canal.

**11. T F A breech birth is the usual presentation of a baby from the birth canal.

**12. T F Having the mother assume a knee-chest position will help take the pressure off a prolapsed cord.

Short Answer

Read each statement or question and write the correct answer or answers in the space provided.

1. In what three ways does slow, deep breathing through the mouth help an expectant mother with labor?

2. What are the four stages of the labor process?

3. What is an indication of an impending delivery?

4. List the two priorities of care for a newborn.

◆ CASE STUDIES

Read the case studies and answer the following questions.

Case 17.1

You have been summoned to a supermarket where a woman has gone into labor. When you arrive, the woman is lying on the floor in pain. You are unsure of whether the baby is crowning. She says this is her first child. She tells you that her labor pains started about an hour ago, but she thought it was only gas. She says also that the baby is not due for another 3 weeks.

1. How long does labor usually take with a first baby?

   a. 4 to 8 hours

   b. 8 to 12 hours

   c. 12 to 24 hours

   d. 24 to 36 hours

2. How many stages of labor are there?

   a. 2

   b. 3

   c. 4

   d. 5

3. Upon examining the woman, you note that the baby is not crowning. What stage of labor is the woman in?

   a. Stage one

   b. Stage two

   c. Stage three

   d. Stage four

4. The first stage of labor ends with complete dilation of the cervix. What happens before the cervix dilates completely?

   a. Crowning occurs.

   b. The placenta is expelled from the uterus.

   c. The baby moves through the birth canal.

   d. Contractions push the baby toward the birth canal.

5. How do you time contractions?

6. What is the average time between contractions just before the birth of the baby?

   a. 60 minutes

   b. 15 to 30 minutes

   c. 5 to 15 minutes

   d. Less than 5 minutes

**Case 17.2

You are called to a home where a woman is in labor. You realize that birth is imminent because you see the baby crowning. You also see a loop of ropelike tissue protruding from the vaginal opening.

1. What complication of childbirth is occurring?

   a. Breech birth

   b. Miscarriage

   c. Prolapsed cord

   d. Abortion

2. Describe what happens in this condition to make it life threatening for the baby.

3. Which of the following is included in the care you should provide for this victim?

   a. Massage the mother's lower abdomen.

   b. Have the mother assume a knee-chest position.

   c. Using a gloved hand, gently prevent the baby's head from coming through the vaginal opening.

   d. Place your index and middle finger of a gloved hand into the vagina to form a "v" around the baby's mouth and nose.

4. T F   Administration of oxygen to the mother is not a normal part of the emergency care for this situation.

◆ SELF-ASSESSMENT

Circle the letter of the best answer.

1. When the baby's head is crowning at the vaginal opening, you should support it by—

   a. Maintaining firm finger pressure against the center of the skull.

   b. Placing your hand lightly on the top of the baby's head.

   c. Placing the palm of your hand firmly against the baby's skull.

   d. Placing one hand on either side of the baby's head.

2. Which of the following questions should you ask to determine whether an expectant mother is in labor and how much time there may be before she delivers?

   1. Is this the first pregnancy?

   2. Has the amniotic sac ruptured?

   3. What are the contractions like?

   4. Has she called her obstetrician or midwife?

   5. Does the mother have the urge to push or bear down?

   a. 1, 3, and 5

   b. 2, 4, and 5

   c. 1, 3, 4, and 5

   d. 1, 2, 3, and 5

3. If you are assisting with a breech delivery, what part of the baby will you see first at the vaginal opening?

   a. Head

   b. Arms

   c. Foot/feet

   d. b or c

4. Which of the following supplies will you need to assist with the delivery of a baby?

   a. Umbilical cord clamps

   b. Sterile water

   c. Clean towels

   d. All of the above

5. If the baby is not crying and/or does not appear to be breathing after delivery, what should you do?

   a. Hold the baby up by its ankles and spank its buttocks.

   b. Suction the baby's throat with the bulb syringe.

   c. Flick the soles of the baby's feet with your fingers.

   d. Administer oxygen by cannula.

6. Which of the following can a woman do to help cope with the pain and discomfort of labor?

   a. Focus on an object in the room while regulating her breathing.

   b. Assume a knee-chest position.

   c. Breathe in and out in a shallow "panting" pattern.

   d. Alternately tense and relax all the muscles in her body.

7. Which of the following is an effective method of controlling persistent vaginal bleeding after a delivery?

   a. Encouraging the baby to nurse

   b. Packing the vagina with a sterile dressing

   c. Firmly massaging the abdomen over the uterus

   d. a and c

8. If you are preparing to assist with the delivery of a baby, what preparations should you make?

   a. Have someone start a large pan of water boiling on the stove.

   b. Place clean sheets, blankets, or towels under the mother's buttocks and over her abdomen.

   c. Get a sterile obstetric kit ready to use in the delivery.

   d. Have the mother lie flat on her back with legs extended.

9. The second stage of labor ends with—

   a. The delivery of the baby.

   b. The dilation of the cervix.

   c. The beginning of contractions.

   d. The delivery of the placenta.

10. How long after delivery of the baby should you expect delivery of the placenta?

    a. 1 hour

    b. Within 30 minutes

    c. Within 24 minutes

    d. Within 10 minutes

Notes

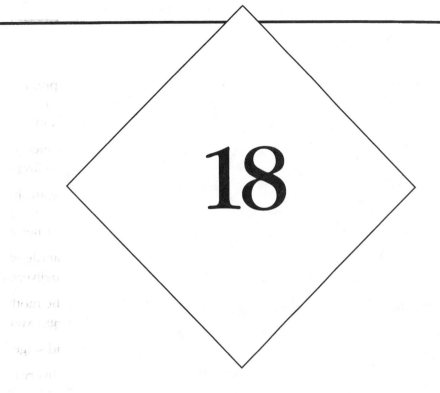

Infants and Children

◆ SUMMARY

Even when uneventful, calls involving infants and children are some of the more stressful situations for first responders. Some of the anxiety occurs because of the lack of experience that rescuers may have in dealing with children. It is important for you to remember that you have learned the skills and knowledge to help you to deal with emergencies, such as airway obstructions, breathing emergencies, circulatory failure, seizures, fever, poisoning, and altered mental status. Most of the principles that you have learned about dealing with adult victims can be applied to infants and children, but you need to remember the differences in infants' and children's developmental characteristics and anatomy.

◆ OUTLINE

◆ LEARNING ACTIVITIES

Matching

Match each term with its definition.
Write its letter on the line in front of the
definition.

Terms

a. Child abuse   e. Febrile seizure

b. Epiglottitis   f. Retraction

c. SIDS   g. Reye's syndrome

d. Child neglect

Definitions

1. _____ An episode of violent muscle
activity brought on by an excessively high fever in an infant or
young child

2. _____ Insufficient attention or respect
given to a child who has a claim
on that attention

3. _____ Physical, psychological, or sexual
assault of a child

4. _____ An illness brought on by high
fever that affects the brain and
other internal organs

5. _____ Bacterial infection that causes
severe inflammation of tissues
above the vocal cords

6. _____ Unexpected death of a seemingly
normal, healthy infant that
occurs during sleep without
evidence of disease

7. _____ A visible sinking-in of soft tissue
between the ribs of an infant
or child

True/False

Circle T if the statement is true; circle F if it is
false.

1. T F   In an emergency, it is not
important to be aware of the
special needs and considerations of infants and children.

2. T F   One of a child's primary
emotions that will affect your
provision of emergency care
is fear.

3. T F   Infants between the ages of 6
months and 1 year old are
relatively easy to approach
and are unlikely to be afraid
of you.

4. T F The most significant anatomical and physiological differences between infants and young children and adults have to do with the airway.

5. T F A normal resting heart rate for an infant, a toddler, and a child are the same as for an adult.

6. T F When opening the airway of an infant or a child, you should tilt the head back only enough to have the victim's nose pointing straight up.

7. T F A sign of a complete airway obstruction in an infant or child who is alert, responsive, and sitting up is the inability to cough, cry, or speak.

8. T F Infants up to 6 months of age often exhibit "stranger anxiety."

9. T F Establishing a good rapport during your care of a child includes reducing anxiety and panic in both the child and the parent or guardian.

10. T F To complete accurate assessments of infants or toddlers, you must place them on a flat, firm surface.

11. T F Most febrile seizures are life threatening.

12. T F For an infant or child with a high fever, administration of aspirin may result in an extremely serious medical condition called Reye's syndrome.

13. T F Your care for a child who is suffering from a high fever is to remove excess clothing and sponge the child with lukewarm water.

14. T F SIDS is a leading cause of death for infants between 1 month and 1 year of age.

15. T F Debriefing after responding to a serious incident involving infants or children should be done with the victim's family.

Short Answer

Read each statement or question and write the correct answer or answers in the space provided.

1. What are five guidelines to use in assessing an ill or injured child?

2. What are three considerations to keep in mind when you are called to assist an ill or injured child?

3. Identify three fears of children.

4. Describe how you would open the airway of an infant or small child.

5. List four possible causes of altered mental status in infants and children.

6. List five signs of child abuse.

7. List two signs of child neglect.

◆ **CASE STUDY**

Read the case study and answer the following questions.

Case 18.1

You are called to the scene of a one-car crash. The driver lost control of the car, and it struck a telephone pole head-on at a high rate of speed. Two adults and an 18-month-old child were in the car when it crashed. The mother is conscious and being cared for by another trained responder. You are providing initial care for the child, who is in a safety seat in the rear seat of the car. You determine that the child is conscious and crying. You see no bleeding or other obvious signs of injury.

1. How should you proceed to care for this victim?

   a. Complete a secondary survey.

   b. Establish rapport with the mother.

   c. Remove the child from the car seat.

   d. Administer supplemental oxygen if you are trained to do so.

2. Which would you expect to be the "normal" pulse rate for a child of this age?

   a. Less than 60 beats per minute

   b. 60 to 100 beats per minute

   c. 100 to 160 beats per minute

   d. Over 160 beats per minute

3. As you perform your assessment, how will your procedure differ from the one you would use with an adult victim?

4. T F To effectively assess and treat this toddler, you should remove him from the child safety seat and let his mother hold him if she is able to do so.

◆ SELF-ASSESSMENT

Circle the letter of the best answer.

1. Which of the following should you do to develop rapport with an injured child?

    a. Talk calmly.

    b. Calm the family as well.

    c. Ask questions that can be easily answered.

    d. All of the above.

2. Which of the following fears of children affects the way you provide care? Fear of—

    a. Cars and trucks.

    b. Peer rejection.

    c. Being touched.

    d. Animals.

3. All of the following are signs of a partial airway obstruction in an infant or child **except**—

    a. Retractions.

    b. Drooling.

    c. Frequent coughing.

    d. Loss of consciousness.

4. Signs of respiratory distress in a child include grunting, respiratory rate greater than 30/40 per minute, use of neck muscles and muscles between and below the margin of the ribs to aid in breathing, and—

    a. Slow or absent heart rate.

    b. Limp muscle tone.

    c. Unresponsiveness.

    d. Flaring of the nostrils.

5. High fever in young children is defined as—

    a. 99 degrees Fahrenheit or above.

    b. 100 degrees Fahrenheit or above.

    c. 101 degrees Fahrenheit or above.

    d. 103 degrees Fahrenheit or above.

6. The normal respiratory rate for preadolescent children is—

    a. 8 to 10 breaths per minute.

    b. 12 to 20 breaths per minute.

    c. 20 to 40 breaths per minute.

    d. 40 to 50 breaths per minute.

7. Which of the following statements about trauma is incorrect?

    a. Injury is the number one cause of death for children in the United States.

    b. The greatest dangers to a child involved in a motor vehicle incident are airway obstruction and bleeding.

    c. The child's head is the least frequently injured part of the child's body.

    d. Children have very soft, pliable ribs that can cause damage and severe internal bleeding.

8. The best position to take in talking to and calming an ill or injured young child is—

    a. At eye level with the child.

    b. At the child's back, out of direct sight.

    c. Standing up so you are above the child.

    d. Holding the child in your arms or on your lap.

9. Which of the following should you do in a case of suspected child abuse?

   a. Confront the parents and ask for an explanation.

   b. Treat the child's injuries without reference to the possible abuse.

   c. Complete an incident report noting your observations and suspicions.

   d. b and c.

10. Prolonged or excessively high fever in a child can result in—

    a. Stroke.

    b. Seizures.

    c. Heart failure.

    d. Breathing difficulty.

Notes

19

EMS Support and Operations

◆ SUMMARY

Depending on the setting in which they work, first responders may or may not have a role in all the nine stages of the EMS response. It is important, however, to understand what happens in each phase:

◆ Preparation
◆ Dispatch
◆ En route to the scene
◆ Arrival at the scene
◆ Transferring the victim to the ambulance
◆ En route to the receiving facility
◆ Arrival at the receiving facility
◆ En route to the station
◆ Post run

As a first responder, you may respond to a multiple casualty incident. A multiple casualty incident is usually managed by an incident commander who appoints other rescuers on the scene to assist in various roles. If many victims are injured or ill, rescue personnel use triage to prioritize care.

At some emergency scenes, victims are trapped in vehicles, and the first responder must gain access to provide care. If you are required to extricate a victim from a vehicle, wear protective equipment, ensure the vehicle is stabilized, and always try simple means of gaining access. Tell victims trapped in vehicles in contact with downed electric wires to remain in the vehicle. Do not approach the vehicle until you know the power has been turned off.

A hazardous materials incident is one in which dangerous chemicals have been released and pose a threat to life. Always stay at a safe distance until the scene is safe to enter.

Any items marked with ** indicate information found only in the Enrichment section of the text.

◆ LEARNING ACTIVITIES

Matching

Match each term with its definition. Write its letter on the line in front of the definition.

Terms

a. Chocking

b. Emergency Medical Dispatcher (EMD)

c. Extrication

d. Hazardous materials (HAZMAT)

e. Hazardous materials incident

f. Incident command system (ICS)

g. Multiple casualty incident (MCI)

h. Packaging

i. Rule of thumb

j. START system

k. Triage

Definitions

1. _____ The removal of a victim trapped in a motor vehicle or in a dangerous situation

2. _____ A method used to control and direct EMS resources at the scene of an emergency

3. _____ A system used at the scene of multiple casualty incidents to quickly assess and prioritize care according to three conditions: breathing, circulation, and level of consciousness

4. _____ Chemical substances that can pose a threat to health, safety, and property

5. _____ Any situation that deals with the unplanned release of dangerous/deadly materials

6. _____ An emergency in which the number of victims may overwhelm the capabilities of a local EMS system

7. _____ Technique used to gauge a safe distance from a hazardous materials site

8. _____ A person who has received special training for giving medical instructions to victims or bystanders before the arrival of more advanced medical personnel

9. _____ The use of wedges against the wheels of a vehicle to help stabilize it

10. _____ The process of sorting and providing care to multiple victims according to the severity of their injuries or illnesses

11. _____ The steps involved in preparing a victim to be moved and moving the victim onto the device to support the victim during transport

True/False

Circle T if the statement is true; circle F if it is false.

1. T F A first responder is a person who has been trained to a maximum standard of care.

2. T F When calling more advanced medical personnel for help, you should tell them your name and the phone number from which you are calling.

3. T F Once you have made a call for help to more advanced medical personnel, you should immediately hang up to keep the phone line clear.

4. T F You should not call more advanced medical personnel for help if the victim asks you not to call.

5. T F Turning on a light switch or using a telephone could create a fire or explosion hazard at a hazardous materials scene.

6. T F Triage is a process that determines the order in which injured victims should be cared for in an emergency.

7. T F An upright vehicle resting on a flat, oily surface should be stabilized by chocking or a similar technique before you try to gain access to the occupants of the vehicle.

8. T F The "rule of thumb" for hazardous materials emergencies says that to be a safe distance away from the site of a hazardous materials spill, you must be far enough away that your thumb, pointing up at arm's length, covers the hazardous area from your view.

9. T   F   Using a center punch or hammer to shatter the glass in a side window should be your first action in attempting to gain access to a victim in a closed, upright vehicle.

10. T   F   A first responder should stabilize an upright vehicle by bracing the vehicle with spare tires, wooden blocks, jacks, or other similar items before attempting to gain access to the occupants.

**11. T   F   There are two kinds of water emergency situations—a swimmer in distress and a drowning person.

**12. T   F   You can help a person in trouble in the water by using reaching and throwing assists.

**13. T   F   You decide to wade into the water to assist a near-drowning victim. You will have a better chance of success if you can reach the victim with your hand rather than with an object like a tree branch or pole.

Short Answer

Read each statement or question and write the correct answer or answers in the space provided.

1. How is a traditional first responder different from a non-traditional first responder?

2. List eight medical supplies that you should include when designing your own first aid kit.

3. List two types of vehicles used in air medical transport.

4. List four ways in which you can reduce the risk of an upright vehicle moving while you are gaining access to and providing emergency care for its occupants?

5. What five clues to the presence of hazardous materials should you be alert for at the scene of an explosion?

◆ CASE STUDY

Read the case study and answer the questions that follow.

Case Study 19.1

You are called to the scene of a car crash in which the car struck and sheared off an electrical pole. The end of a severed wire rests on top of the car. A driver and a passenger are in the car when you arrive. You call through an open window; the driver is unresponsive. The passenger, a woman, tells you that the driver, her husband, was complaining of chest pain just before the crash and seemed to lose control of the car. She says she is unhurt and pleads with you to get them out of the car and help her husband.

1. What is your first priority in responding to this situation?

    a. Calling the power company for assistance

    b. Establishing a safety zone around the car for yourself and bystanders

    c. Pulling or pushing the wire carefully from the car with a nonmetal pole

    d. Telling the woman in the car to carefully open her door and be prepared to jump clear.

2. If you are unable to safely gain access to the driver, what should you do while waiting for the power company?

    a. Tell the woman to jump clear of the car, being careful not to touch the car or wire while doing so.

    b. Instruct the woman on how to determine whether her husband is breathing and how to check his pulse.

    c. Look carefully at the wire to see if it is "live."

    d. b and c.

3. T   F   A safe distance away from the car is half the distance between the two poles from which the severed wire was strung.

4. Once you gain access to the driver and his wife, what four signs and symptoms would you watch out for to determine whether either one has an electrical injury?

◆ SELF-ASSESSMENT

Circle the letter of the best answer.

1. The phase of a call that involves using body substance isolation before approaching the victim, and observing the scene for hazards, mechanism of the injury or nature of the illness, and the need additional help is—

    a. Preparing for an Emergency Call.

    b. En-Route to the Scene.

    c. Arrival at the Scene.

    d. Transferring the Victim to the Ambulance.

2. The phase of a call in which crew members complete whatever documentation is necessary to meet local or state standards and their organization's protocols is—

    a. En-Route to the Receiving Facility.

    b. At the Receiving Facility.

    c. En-Route to the Station.

    d. Post Run.

3. The leadership positions in an Incident Command System (ICS) include all of the following except—

a. Transportation section officer.

b. Operations section officer.

c. Planning section officer.

d. Logistics section officer.

4. In surveying the scene, you note a Department of Transportation-type placard on the rear door of the truck indicating the presence of hazardous materials. What information should you look for on the placard?

a. The name, color, and/or identifying number of the materials in the truck

b. The amount of chemicals usually in the truck

c. The name and telephone number of the manufacturer of the stored chemicals

d. All the above

5. An emergency that may overwhelm the capabilities of the local EMS system is called—

a. Triage.

b. A multiple casualty incident.

c. An incident command system.

d. Simple Triage and Rapid Treatment.

6. Which of the following could indicate the presence of hazardous materials?

a. Unusual odors

b. Clouds of vapor

c. Downed wires

d. a and b

7. A system used to control and direct resources at the scene of an emergency is called the—

a. Incident command system.

b. Triage system.

c. Multiple casualty system.

d. Emergency control system.

8. At the scene of a tanker truck crash, you note a placard on the side of the truck. What information about the materials in the tanker would you expect to find on the placard?

a. The name and identifying number of the substance

b. Whether the chemical is explosive, flammable, corrosive, or radioactive

c. The amount of chemical carried in the tanker

d. a and b

9. At the scene of a single car collision in which a car has hit a telephone pole and a wire is lying on top of the car, your first priority is to—

a. Immediately remove the occupants from the car.

b. Remove the wire from the car.

c. Ensure your safety and that of any bystanders.

d. Stabilize the car to prevent it from moving.

10. You are deciding whether to attempt to pull a victim away from a car that has smoke coming from the hood. Which of the following will help you make the decision?

    a. The victim weighs about 40 pounds less than you.

    b. There are no bystanders willing to help.

    c. The area around the victim is damp with gas.

    d. All of the above.

**11. A woman is struggling in the water at the deep end of a swimming pool. In attempting a rescue, which is the appropriate way to reach her and pull her to the side of the pool?

    a. Lie down at the side of the pool, and reach to her with your arm.

    b. Enter the water, and extend your hand or foot to her.

    c. Remove your shoes, and jump in to assist her to the side.

    d. Call for help, and wade toward the deep end to reach her.

Notes

Notes

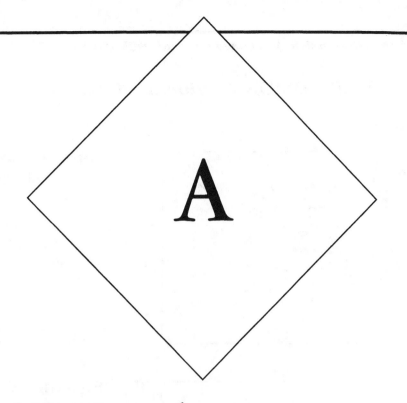

Automated External Defibrillation (AED)

PRACTICE SESSION: *Automated External Defibrillation (AED)*

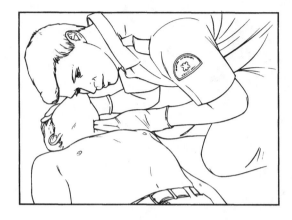

☐ **Confirm cardiac arrest**
  ◆ Check pulse for 5–10 seconds.

If no pulse… begin CPR until AED is attached to victim.

If pulse… check for breathing

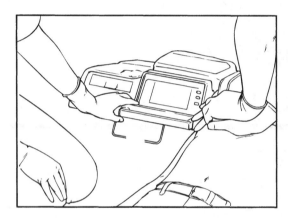

☐ **Turn on the AED**
  ◆ If AED has a voice recorder, give a verbal report that includes:
    ◆ Your identity and location.
    ◆ Assessment findings
    ◆ Any significant events

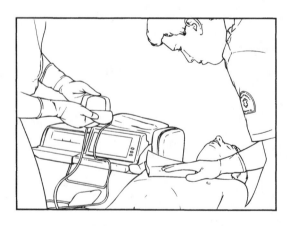

☐ **Attach the device**
  ◆ Wipe the chest dry.
  ◆ Connect cables to pads, if necessary. Place pads on victim's chest.
    ◆ Right pad goes on the right side between the nipple and the collarbone.
    ◆ Left pad goes on the left side below the nipple.

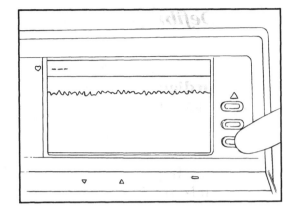

Press analyze button

◆ Make sure no one is touching the victim.
◆ Press the button marked "Analyze."

If shock is indicated...

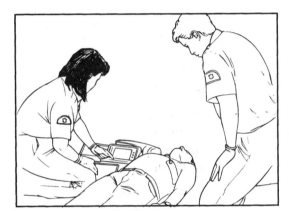

Deliver shock

◆ If the AED identifies a shockable rhythm, prepare to deliver shock.
◆ Instruct others to "stand clear."
◆ Push the shock button to defibrillate.

After delivering the shock, press the analyze button again. Deliver another shock if indicated. Total number of shocks delivered is determined by local protocols.

If no shock is indicated...

◆ Recheck pulse and start CPR.
◆ After 1 minute of CPR analyze again.

Notes

Answers to Exercises

Unit 1

Matching: 1. c; 2. e; 3. a; 4. h; 5. i; 6. b; 7. d; 8. f; 9. j; 10. g. True/False: 1. F; 2. T; 3. T; 4. F; 5. T; 6. T; 7. T; 8. T; 9. T. Short Answer: 1. a. Citizen response; b. Early activation of EMS; c. First responder care; d. Advanced prehospital care; e. Hospital care; f. Rehabilitation. 2. Maintaining a caring and professional attitude; controlling your own fears; presenting a professional appearance; keeping your skills and knowledge up to date; staying fit with daily exercise and a healthy diet; maintaining a healthy lifestyle. 3. It created the National Highway Traffic Safety Administration (NHTSA) within the Department of Transportation (DOT), and created a multi-tiered, nationwide system of emergency health care. 4. Regulation and Policy, Resource Management, Human Resources and Training, Transportation, Facilities, Communications, Public Information and Education, Medical Oversight, Trauma Systems, and Evaluation. 5. Direct and indirect medical control are the same because both are a kind of medical oversight. Direct medical control is when the physician speaks directly with emergency care providers at the scene of an emergency. Indirect medical control is physician oversight which includes education, protocol review, and quality improvement of emergency care providers. Self-Assessment: 1. a; 2. c; 3. b; 4. c; 5. d; 6. b; 7. a; 8. b; 9. d; 10. b.

Unit 2

Matching: 1. b; 2. d; 3. c; 4. a; 5. e. **Matching: 1. c; 2. b; 3. e; 4. a; 5. d;. True/False: 1. T; 2. F; 3. F; 4. T; 5. F; 6. F; 7. T; 8. F; 9. T; 10. F; 11. T; 12. F; 13. T; 14. F; 15. T; 16. F; 17. T; 18. F; 19. F. Short Answer: 1. Mass casualty incident; trauma in infants and children; injuries caused by trauma. 2. Anxiety; denial/disbelief; anger; bargaining; guilt/depression; acceptance. 3. Recognize that the victim's needs include dignity, respect, sharing, communication, privacy, and control; allow family members to express rage, anger, and despair; listen empathetically; do not falsely reassure; use a gentle tone of voice; let the victim know that everything that can be done to help will be done; use a reassuring touch, if it is appropriate; comfort the family. 4. Multiple casualties; rescues; emergencies involving children; failed resuscitation attempts; death or serious injury to co-workers. 5. Location of the emergency; extent of the emergency; apparent scene dangers; number of victims; behavior of bystanders. 6. Signs or placards; clouds of vapor; spilled liquids or solids; unusual odors; leaking containers, bottles, or cylinders; chemical transport tanks or containers. 7. To protect an injured person; to protect any rescuers, including yourself; to warn oncoming traffic if the situation is not clearly visible. 8. a. Do not enter the scene until summoned by law enforcement personnel; b. Do not attempt a rescue until wreckage has been stabilized; c. Do not enter until summoned by law enforcement personnel. Do not touch anyone except who you must give care to. **d. Unsafe structures. **e. Multiple victims. **9. Making every effort to understand fully what the victim is trying to say; repeating back to the victim, in your own words, what he or she said; avoiding criticism or rejection of the victim's statements; using open-ended questions such as, "You appear to be very sad," or "What problems are you having?"; generally, avoiding questions that can be answered with "yes" or "no." 10. Live electrical wires; hazardous materials; flames; shattered glass; passing traffic; fumes; unstable telephone poles; spilled container; leaking gasoline. Case Study: 2. 1. 1. Cover the victim and protect her from any unnecessary exposure; clear the area of any bystanders, except those friends or family able to help provide emotional support; do not disrupt the crime scene by handling items unrelated to the victim's care; summon more advanced medical personnel and law enforcement personnel; do not remove any clothing unless it is absolutely necessary to provide care for injuries; care for any physical injuries; discourage the victim from bathing, showering, or douching prior to a medical examination; do not question the victim about the specifics of the assault. 2. F; 3. T. **Case Study 2.2. 1. c; 2. F; 3. a; 4. F. Self-Assessment: 1. d; 2. a; 3. a; 4. b; 5. a; 6. c; 7. d; 8. d; 9. c; 10. d; 11. b; 12. d; 13. d; 14. a; 15. c.

Unit 3 Answers

Matching: 1. b; **2.** d; **3.** e; **4.** a; **5.** c; **6.** g ; **7.** f. **True/False: 1.** F; **2.** T; **3.** F; **4.** F; **5.** T; **6.** F; **7.** T; **8.** F; **9.** F; **10.** F; **11.** T; **12.** T. **Short Answer: 1.** A pathogen; the pathogen is in sufficient quantity to cause disease; a person is vulnerable to the pathogen; the pathogen is transmitted through the correct entry site. **2.** A solution of $^1/_4$ cup of common household chlorine bleach in a gallon of water. **3.** Direct and indirect contact; air borne, direct contact with body fluids; direct contact; airborne, direct and indirect contact; direct and indirect contact. **4.** Wear disposable gloves; wash hands thoroughly after providing care; use resuscitation devices; clean and disinfect all equipment and work surfaces possibly contaminated by blood or other body fluids; wear protective coverings, such as a mask, eyewear, and gown; place sharp items in puncture resistant containers; discard gloves that are peeling, discolored, torn, or punctured; change gloves between contacts, and avoid handling items; cover any cuts, scrapes, or skin irritations you may have by wearing protective clothing and/or bandages; avoid eating, drinking, and touching your mouth, nose, or eyes while providing care or before washing hands; avoid needle stick injuries by not attempting to bend or recap any needles; place all contaminated clothing in well marked plastic bags for disposal or washing; getting immunizations for DPT, Hepatitis B, MMR, influenza, and varicella. **Case Study 3.1: 1.** d; **2.** F; **3.** Rabies; **4.** a. **Case Study 3.2: 1.** Protocols/standard procedures; **2.** T; **3.** T. **Self-Assessment: 1.** c; **2.** d; **3.** b; **4.** a; **5.** c; **6.** d; **7.** b; **8.** d; **9.** a; **10.** c; **11.** d.

Unit 4

Matching: 1. f; **2.** c; **3.** a; **4.** d; **5.** i; **6.** g; **7.** e; **8.** h; **9.** b. ****Matching: 1.** c; **2.** a; **3.** d; **4.** b. **True/False: 1.** F; **2.** F; **3.** T; **4.** F; **5.** T; **6.** F; **7.** T; **8.** T; **9.** F; ****10.** T; ****11.** F; ****12.** T; ****13.** F; ****14.** F; ****15.** T; ****16.** F. **Short Answer: 1.** Expressed consent is the permission granted to you to care for a victim after you have clearly identified yourself, given your level of training, explained what you think may be wrong, and explained what you plan to do; implied consent is the assumed permission granted to you to care for a victim who is unconscious or, in your best judgment, is confused, mentally impaired, or seriously ill or injured; in these cases, the law assumes that the person would give consent for care if he or she were able to do so.

2. Duty, breach, cause, and damage. ****3.** Visually impaired; hearing impaired; physically disabled; developmentally disabled. **Case Study 4.1: 1.** There is no legal duty to act in this situation because you are not at work or on duty; however, you may feel that you have a moral duty to act.; **2.** d; **3.** Traffic; spilled gasoline; untrained bystanders trying to help; and, possibly, hazardous materials; **4.** F. ****Case Study 4.2: 1.** T; **2.** c. ****Case Study 4.3: 1.** Sign language; lip reading; writing messages on paper. **2.** F. **Self-Assessment: 1.** b; **2.** c; **3.** c; **4.** b; **5.** d; **6.** c; **7.** a; ****8.** b; ****9.** b; ****10.** d.

Unit 5

Matching: 1. d; **2.** a; **3.** c; **4.** b; **5.** e. ****Matching: 1.** b; **2.** c; **3.** a; **4.** e; **5.** d. **True/False: 1.** F; **2.** F; **3.** T; **4.** F; **5.** T; **6.** T; **7.** T; **8.** F; **9.** T; **10.** F; **11.** F; **12.** T. **Short Answer: 1. a.** Cranial; **b.** Spinal; **c.** Thoracic; **d.** Abdominal; **e.** Pelvic. **2. a.** Brain; **b.** Spinal cord; **c.** Heart and lungs; **d.** liver, pancreas, intestines, stomach, kidneys, and spleen; **e.** Bladder, rectum, and female reproductive organs. **3. a.** Epiglottis; **b.** esophagus; **c.** Lungs; **d.** Trachea. ****4.** Standing facing front, arms at side, palms facing to the front. **Case Study 5.1: **1.** Distal; Proximal. ****2.** Anterior; ****3.** Lateral; **4.** c. **Case Study 5.2: 1.** c; **2.** T; **3.** Glands; **4.** To release fluid and other substances into the blood or onto the skin; **5.** Hormones. **Self-Assessment: 1.** b; **2.** a; **3.** a; **4.** a; **5.** c; **6.** a; **7.** b; **8.** a; **9.** d; **10.** b.

Unit 6

Matching: 1. d; **2.** a; **3.** e; **4.** c; **5.** b. **True/False: 1.** F; **2.** T; **3.** F; **4.** T; **5.** T; **6.** T; **7.** T; **8.** F; **9.** T; **10.** T. **Short Answer: 1.** There is immediate danger to the rescuer or the victim. You need to gain access to a more seriously injured victim. You cannot provided proper care without moving the victim. **2.** The distance the victim must be moved; dangerous conditions at the scene; the size of the victim; your physical ability; whether others can help you; the victim's condition; any aids to transport at the scene. **3.** Immediate danger, gaining access to other victims; providing proper care. **4.** Assists, carries, drags. **Case Study 6. 1.** The danger of smoke and/or fire; the size of the victim; your physical ability; the availability of others to help; the victim's injuries. **2.** c. **Self-Assessment: 1.** b; **2.** d; **3.** d; **4.** c; **5.** a; **6.** b; **7.** c; **8.** b; **9.** d; **10.** c.

Unit 7

Matching: **1.** e; **2.** b; **3.** a; **4.** f; **5.** d; **6.** c. ****Matching 1.** e; **2.** b; **3.** a; **4.** d; **5.** c. **True/False**: **1.** F; **2.** F; **3.** F; **4.** T; **5.** F; **6.** T; **7.** F; **8.** T; **9.** F; **10.** T; **11.** T; **12.** T; **13.** F; **14.** T; **15.** F; **16.** F; **17.** T. **Short Answer**: **1.** Scene size-up; perform an initial assessment; perform a physical exam; obtain a SAMPLE history; perform an ongoing assessment. **2.** Scene safety; the mechanism of injury/nature of illness; the number of victims; the resources needed. **3.** Forming a general impression; assess the level of consciousness; assess the airway, breathing, and circulation. **4.** Alert; verbal; painful; unresponsive. **5.** A systematic head-to-toe examination that gathers additional information about injuries or medical problems. **6.** Signs and symptoms; allergies; medications; pertinent past history; last oral intake; events leading up to the incident. **7.** Stethoscope and blood pressure cuff. **8.** 110/70. **Case Study 7.1**: **1.** c; **2.** b; **3.** Blood pressure, level of consciousness, capillary refill. **Case Study 7.2**: **1.** d; **2.** a; **3.** Deformity, open injuries, tenderness, swelling. **Self-Assessment**: **1.** c; **2.** d; **3.** a; **4.** b; **5.** d; **6.** d; **7.** c; **8.** d; **9.** d; **10.** c.

Unit 8

Matching: **1.** e; **2.** c; **3.** b; **4.** a; **5.** d; **6.** f. **True/False**: **1.** F; **2.** T; **3.** F; **4.** T; **5.** T; **6.** T; **7.** T; **8.** F; **9.** F; **10.** F; **11.** T; **12.** T; **13.** F; **14.** T; **15.** F. **Short Answer**: **1.** The victim begins to breathe; the victim has no pulse; you begin CPR; another rescuer of equal or greater training takes over; you are too exhausted to continue; the scene becomes unsafe. **2.** Swallowing large pieces of poorly chewed food; drinking alcohol before meals; wearing dentures; eating while talking excitedly or laughing or eating too fast; walking, playing, or running with food or objects in the mouth. **3.** Slow or rapid breathing; unusually deep or shallow breaths; gasping for breath; wheezing, gurgling, or making high-pitched noises; unusually moist skin; flushed, pale or ashen, or bluish skin; shortness of breath; dizziness or light headedness; pain in the chest, tingling in hands and feet. **4. a.** 4, Give quick upward thrusts into the abdomen; **b.** 2, Stand behind the victim and wrap your arms around him or her; **c.** 1, Determine if the person is choking; **d.** 3, Make a fist with one of your hands; place the thumb side of your fist against the victim's abdomen just above the navel. **5. a.** 4, Deliver 5 back blows; **b.** 6, Do a finger sweep if you see the object; **c.** 2, Give 2 slow breaths; **d.** 5, Deliver 5 chest thrusts;

e. 1, Open the airway and check for breathing. **f.** 3, Retilt the head and repeat breaths. **Case Study 8.1**: **1.** d; **2.** Facedown on your forearm while providing back blows; face up along your forearm while administering chest thrusts. **3.** F; **4.** Place the pad of your ring finger on the infant's breastbone just under the nipple line. Place the pads of the middle and index fingers on the infant's breastbone under the nipple line. Raise the ring finger off her chest. **5.** T. **Case Study 8.2**: **1.** c; **2.** d; **3.** Turn the victim's head and body to the side as a unit; wipe the mouth clean; reposition the victim, moving him as a unit, and continue rescue breathing. **4.** F; **5.** Once a minute. **6.** b. **Self-Assessment**: **1.** c; **2.** b; **3.** d; **4.** c; **5.** c; **6.** d; **7.** d; **8.** a; **9.** d; **10.** c.

Unit 9

Matching: **1.** b; **2.** c; **3.** d; **4.** a; **5.** e. ****Matching 1.** a; **2.** b; **3.** c; **4.** e; **5.** d. **True/False**: **1.** T; **2.** F; **3.** T; **4.** T; **5.** F; **6.** F; **7.** F; **8.** T; **9.** F; **10.** T; **11.** F; **12.** T; **13.** T; **14.** F; **15.** T; **16.** T; **17.** F; **18.** F; **19.** T; **20.** T. **Short Answer**: **1.** Tilt the victim's head back; lift the victim's jaw with both hands; keep the victim's mouth open with your thumbs. **2.** Turn the head to the side; open the mouth; remove large debris; measure the device; insert the device; suction as you remove the tip for no more than 15 seconds. **3.** Oxygen cylinder; pressure regulator with flowmeter; delivery device. **4.** Do not operate around open flame or sparks; do not stand the cylinder upright unless it is secured; do not use grease, oil, or petroleum products on the pressure regulator; always check to see that oxygen is flowing before placing a device on a person's face. **5.** Green color; yellow-diamond symbol with word "Oxidizer"; three holes in the cylinder valve allowing for the attachment of only an oxygen pressure regulator. **Case Study 9.1**: **1.** F; **2.** Measure from the victim's earlobe to the corner of the mouth; **3.** b; **4.** d. **Case Study 9.2**: **1.** T; **2.** T; **3.** c. **Self-Assessment**: **1.** c; **2.** a; **3.** c; **4.** a; **5.** d; **6.** c; **7.** d; **8.** b; **9.** c; **10.** a.

Unit 10

Matching: **1.** c; **2.** e; **3.** b; **4.** a; **5.** g; **6.** d; **7.** f. **Matching Cycle**: **1.** c; **2.** b; **3.** a. **True/False**: **1.** T; **2.** T; **3.** F; **4.** T; **5.** F; **6.** F; **7.** T; **8.** F; **9.** T; **10.** T; **11.** F; **12.** T; **13.** T; **14.** F; **15.** T; **16.** T; **17.** F; **18.** T; **19.** F; **20.** F. **Short Answer**: **1.** When did the pain start? What brought it on? Does anything lessen it? What does it feel like? Where does it hurt? **2.** Another trained person takes over for you; advanced medical personnel arrive and take over; you are exhausted and unable to continue; the scene suddenly becomes unsafe; the victim's heart starts beating; a defibrillator is able to be used; a valid DNR order is presented. **3.** Slide the middle finger and index finger up the edge of the ribs to the notch at the base of the sternum; position the heel of your other hand on the sternum, place your other hand on top; apply pressure with the heel of your hand and with the fingers off the chest. **4.** Agitation; drowsiness; change in skin color; increased difficulty breathing; increased heart and breathing rates. **5.** When CPR is not being given, and 2 or more rescuers arrive at the same time; one rescuer is giving CPR, and a second is available to begin two-rescuer CPR; one rescuer tires and rescuers change positions. **Case Study 10.1**: **1.** F; **2.** a; **3.** T; **4.** T; **5.** After 1 minute. **6.** T. **Case Study 10.2**: **1.** a; **2.** F; **3.** Inquire about chest pain; inquire about any history of heart disease and about medications the victim might be taking; administer oxygen if available and if you are trained to do so; calm and reassure the victim; monitor vital signs. **4.** Most people who die from heart attacks do so within 1 to 2 hours of experiencing the first symptoms. **Case Study 10.3**: **1.** b; **2.** c; **3.** Find the nipples; place index finger on the sternum just below an imaginary line between the nipples; place pads of next two fingers on the sternum next to the index finger; raise the index finger off the chest—avoid pressure on the notch of the sternum. **4.** T; **5.** 5 compressions followed by 1 breath. **Self-Assessment**: **1.** a; **2.** d; **3.** d; **4.** b; **5.** d; **6.** a; **7.** d; **8.** b; **9.** c; **10.** a.

Unit 11

Matching: **1.** b; **2.** h; **3.** e; **4.** f; **5.** g; **6.** c; **7.** a; **8.** d; **9.** j; **10.** i. **True/False**: **1.** F; **2.** T; **3.** T; **4.** F; **5.** T; **6.** T; **7.** F; **8.** T; **9.** F; **10.** F; **11.** T; **12.** F; **13.** F; **14.** F; **15.** F; **16.** T; **17.** F; **18.** F; **19.** T. **Short Answer**: **1.** Transporting oxygen, nutrients, and wastes; protecting against disease by producing antibodies and defending against germs; helping maintain constant body temperature by circulating throughout the body. **2.** Blood spurting from a wound; blood that does not clot after you have taken all available measures to control bleeding. **3.** Bruising; tender, swollen, or firm soft tissue; anxiety or restlessness; rapid, weak pulse; rapid breathing; cool, moist skin; pale or bluish skin; nausea and vomiting; excessive thirst; declining level of consciousness; drop

in blood pressure. **4.** Apply direct pressure; elevate the injured area; apply a pressure bandage; apply pressure at a pressure point. **5.** Restlessness and irritability. **6.** Control external bleeding; elevate the legs about 12 inches; administer oxygen if it is available and you are trained to do so; do not give anything by mouth; summon more advanced medical personnel. **7.** The heart must be working well; an adequate amount of blood must be circulating in the body; the blood vessels must be intact and be able to adjust to blood flow. **Case Study 11.1**: **1.** d; **2.** F; **3.** Monitor ABCs and vital signs; help victim rest in the most comfortable position; maintain normal body temperature; reassure victim; provide care for other conditions; administer oxygen if it is available and you are trained to do so. **Case Study 11.2**: **1.** T; **2.** d; **3.** a. **Case Study 11.3**: **1.** d; **2.** b; **3.** d. **Self-Assessment**: **1.** b; **2.** c; **3.** b; **4.** d; **5.** a; **6.** d; **7.** c; **8.** a; **9.** d; **10.** b; **11.** b; **12.** d.

Unit 12

Matching: **1.** e; **2.** l; **3.** m; **4.** h; **5.** k; **6.** d; **7.** f; **8.** g; **9.** a; **10.** c; **11.** b; **12.** j; **13.** i; **14.** n. **True/False**: **1.** F; **2.** T; **3.** F; **4.** F; **5.** T; **6.** F; **7.** F; **8.** T; **9.** T; **10.** F; **11.** T; **12.** T; **13.** T; **14.** F; **15.** T; **16.** T; **17.** T; **18.** F; **19.** F; **20.** T. **Short Answer**: **1.** Do not remove the object; use bulky dressings to stabilize the object; control any bleeding by bandaging the dressings in place around the object. **2.** Temperature of the burn source; length of exposure to the source; location of the burn; extent of the burn; victim's age and medical condition. **3.** Cool and cover burns to reduce pain; place the victim lying down unless it causes breathing difficulty; elevate the burned areas. above the level of the heart; maintain normal body temperature and prevent chilling; administer oxygen if it is available, it is safe to do so, and you are trained to use it. **4.** Abrasion; laceration; avulsion; puncture. **5.** Do not wash the wound; control bleeding with direct pressure and elevation; apply a pressure bandage; summon more advanced medical personnel; use a pressure point if necessary; wash hands immediately after completing care. **Case Study 12.1**: **1.** F; **2.** F; **3.** d; **4.** c; **Case Study 12.2**: **1.** d; **2.** Use cool water until the areas around the burns are not warm to the touch. Do **not** use ice or ice water. **3.** F; **4.** d; **5.** T; **6.** b. **Case Study 12.3**: **1.** c; **2.** F; **3.** d. **Self-Assessment**: **1.** a; **2.** b; **3.** c; **4.** a; **5.** b; **6.** d; **7.** a; **8.** b; **9.** d; **10.** d.

Unit 13

Matching: 1. d; **2.** c; **3.** b; **4.** a; **5.** e. ****Matching: 1.** d; **2.** a; **3.** g; **4.** e; **5.** b; **6.** h; **7.** c; **8.** f. **True/False: 1.** T; **2.** F; **3.** F; **4.** T; **5.** T; **6.** F; **7.** F; **8.** T; **9.** F; **10.** F; **11.** F; **12.** T; **13.** T; **14.** T; **15.** F; **16.** T; ****17.** T; ****18.** F; ****19.** F; ****20.** T; ****21.** T; ****22.** T; ****23.** T; ****24.** F; ****25.** T. **Short Answer: 1.** Splint only if you can do so without causing more pain and discomfort to the victim; splint an injury in the position that you find it; splint the injury site and the joints above and below it; check areas above and below the splint for proper circulation and sensation before and after splinting. **2.** Cold helps reduce swelling and eases pain and discomfort. **3.** Pain and tenderness; swelling; grating; deformity or angulation; bruising (discoloration); exposed bone ends; joint locked into position. **4.** Direct force; indirect force; twisting force. **5.** Lessens pain; prevents further damage to soft tissues; reduces the risk of serious bleeding; reduces the possibility of loss of circulation to the injured part; prevents a closed painful, swollen, deformed extremity injury from becoming an open painful, swollen, deformed extremity injury. **6.** Place one long padded splint on the outside of the leg from above the hip to beyond the foot; place s shorter padded splint on the inside of the leg extending beyond the foot; secure the splints with cravats. **7.** Pain in the joint; tenderness; moderate or severe swelling; discoloration; significant deformity; inability to move or use the affected part; severe external bleeding. **8.** Check before splinting to help determine if the injury has impaired blood flow or nerve function; check after splinting to assure that splinting did not cause impairment of circulation or nerve function; loosen splint if it has done either or both. ****9. a.** Collarbone; **b.** Humerus; **c.** Radius; **d.** Ulna; **e.** Femur; **f.** Patella; **g.** Fibula; **h.** Tibia. **Case Study 13.1: 1.** b; **2.** F; **3.** b; **4.** Loosen the splint and recheck circulation. **Case Study 13.2: 1.** T; **2.** a; **3.** Splint and elevate the injured part and apply a cold pack. **4.** Check for a radial pulse; feel the hand for warmth; check to determine if the victim can feel you touching his hand. **Case Study 13.3: 1.** T; **2.** c; **3.** T; **4.** Control external bleeding, if any; immobilize the ankles; secure splints with cravats or roller bandage; apply ice or cold packs to the ankles/feet; call more advanced medical personnel and keep the victim from moving. ****Case Study 13.4: 1.** c; **2.** T; **3.** Moving from a cold to a warm area causes the air in the splint to expand, making the splint tighter; moving from a warm area to a colder area can cause the splint to loosen. **4.** T. **Self-Assessment: 1.** d; **2.** b; **3.** d; **4.** b; **5.** a; **6.** b; **7.** a; **8.** d; **9.** a; **10.** b; ****11.** a; ****12.** c; ****13.** c; ****14.** a; ****15.** d; ****16.** b. ****17.** d; ****18.** c; ****19.** b.

Unit 14

Matching: 1. g; **2.** a; **3.** c; **4.** b; **5.** d; **6.** f; **7.** e . **True/False: 1.** F; **2.** F; **3.** F; **4.** T; **5.** T; **6.** F; **7.** T; **8.** T; **9.** F; **10.** T; **11.** F; **12.** T; **13.** F; **14.** F; **15.** F; **16.** T. **Short Answer: 1.** The head is severely angled to one side; the victim complains of pain, pressure, or muscle spasm in the neck as you try to move the head; you feel resistance when attempting to move the head. **2.** You cannot control bleeding; the bleeding stops and then recurs; the bleeding is a result of high blood pressure. **3.** A fall from a height greater than the victim's height; any diving mishap; a person found unconscious for unknown reasons; any injury involving severe blunt force to the head or trunk; any penetrating injury to the head or trunk; a motor vehicle crash involving victims not wearing safety belts or that results in a broken windshield or deformed steering wheel; a person thrown from a motor vehicle; any injury in which a victim's helmet is broken; any incident involving a lightning strike; any person found unconscious in water 5 feet deep or less. **4.** Place the victim on his or her back; do not remove the object; place a sterile dressing around the object; place a covering (such as a cup) over the eye to prevent pressure on the eyeball; apply a bandage. **5.** Changes in level of consciousness; pain or pressure; tingling or loss of sensation; partial or complete loss of movement; unusual bumps or depressions; blood or other fluids draining from the ears or nose; profuse external bleeding of the head, neck, or back; seizures; impaired breathing or vision from injury; nausea or vomiting; persistent headache; loss of balance; bruising around eyes or behind ears; combative or aggressive behavior. **6.** Apply in-line stabilization; apply a cervical collar; log-roll the victim onto a backboard; secure the victim's body; secure the victim's head. **7.** Wear safety belts; wear approved helmets, eyewear, face guards, and mouth guards; prevent falls; obey rules; avoid inappropriate use of drugs; inspect equipment periodically;

think and talk about safety. **Case Study 14.1: 1.** c; **2.** Blood from a ruptured vessel in the brain can accumulate in the skull; there is little empty space in the skull, so bleeding can create pressure. **3.** b; **4.** d; **5.** T. **Case Study 14.2: 1.** c; **2.** Place a rolled sterile dressing in the space left by the missing teeth; have the victim bite down on the dressing; **3.** F; **4.** b. **Self-Assessment: 1.** d; **2.** b; **3.** d; **4.** a; **5.** c; **6.** c; **7.** d; **8.** b; **9.** d.

Unit 15

Matching: 1. e; **2.** a; **3.** d; **4.** b; **5.** c. ****Matching 1.** b; **2.** a; **3.** c; **4.** e; **5.** d. **True/False: 1.** T; **2.** F; **3.** F; **4.** F; **5.** F; **6.** T; **7.** F; **8.** T; **9.** T; **10.** F; **11.** F; **12.** F; **13.** F; **14.** T; **15.** T; **16.** T; **17.** F; **18.** F; **19.** F; **20.** T. **Short Answer: 1.** Changes in a victim's level of consciousness; light headedness, dizziness, and weakness; nausea; vomiting; changes in breathing, pulse, and skin color. **2.** Prevent further harm; monitor the vital signs; summon more advanced medical personnel; help the victim rest comfortably; maintain normal body temperature; provide reassurance; administer oxygen if available. **3.** Seizure lasts more than a few minutes; victim has repeated seizures; victim appears to be injured; victim is pregnant; victim is a known diabetic; victim is an infant or child; seizure takes place in water; uncertain about the cause of the seizure; victim fails to regain consciousness after the seizure. **4.** A first responder does not need to determine the precise cause of a medical emergency. Knowing and following the basic principles of care are all that is needed. **5.** Fever; infection; poisoning; high or low blood sugar; head injury; conditions resulting in decreased blood flow or oxygen to the brain; conditions resulting from mental, emotional, or behavioral disorders. **Case Study 15.1: 1.** d; **2.** Numbness; white, waxy extremity; **3.** c; **4.** T. **Case Study 15.2: 1.** d; **2.** question food and medication intake, as well as any present illness; **3.** Cease activity; place in position of comfort; if not nauseated, give cool water; provide sugar for the possible diabetic problem. Case 15.3 **1.** c; **2.** b; **3.** b; **4.** d. **Self-Assessment: 1.** d; **2.** d; **3.** b; **4.** d; **5.** d; **6.** c; **7.** a; **8.** d; **9.** b; **10.** d.

Unit 16

Matching: 1. k; **2.** a; **3.** f; **4.** d; **5.** j; **6.** g; **7.** c; **8.** i; **9.** b; **10.** h; **11.** e. **True/False: 1.** F; **2.** T; **3.** F; **4.** T; **5.** T; **6.** F; **7.** T; **8.** T; **9.** F; **10.** F; **11.** T; **12.** T; **13.** T; **14.** T; **15.** F;

16. T; **17.** T; **18.** F; **19.** F; **20.** F. **Short Answer: 1.** Do not apply ice. Do not cut the wound. Do not apply a tourniquet. Do not use electric shock. **2.** What type of poison was taken? How much was taken? When was it taken? **3.** Injection; inhalation; ingestion; absorption. **4.** Swelling and reddening skin; hives; itching; dizziness; weakness; vomiting; nausea; difficulty breathing; rash. **5.** Approximately 1/2 to 1 bottle (12.5 - 25 grams). **Case Study 16.1: 1.** d; **2.** Bites from a tick infected with a disease take several days or more to cause symptoms. **3.** c; **4.** T; **5.** b. **Case Study 16.2: 1.** F; **2.** T; **3.** d; **4.** c. **Self-Assessment: 1.** d; **2.** a; **3.** c; **4.** d; **5.** d; **6.** a; **7.** c; **8.** a; **9.** d; **10.** b.

Unit 17

Matching: 1. j; **2.** i; **3.** g; **4.** c; **5.** f; **6.** h; **7.** a; **8.** d; **9.** e; **10.** b; ****Matching: 1.** b; **2.** a; **3.** c. **True/False: 1.** T; **2.** T; **3.** T; **4.** F; **5.** T; **6.** F; **7.** T; **8.** T; **9.** F; **10.** F; ****11.** F; ****12.** T. **Short Answer: 1.** Aids muscle relaxation; offers a distraction from the pain; ensures adequate oxygen to both the mother and the baby during labor. **2.** Stage one—Preparation; Stage two—Delivery of the baby; Stage three—Delivery of the placenta; Stage four—Stabilization. **3.** The mother feels the urge to push or feels as if she needs to have a bowel movement. **4.** Check to see if the airway is open and clear. Maintain normal body temperature. **Case Study 17.1: 1.** c; **2.** c; **3.** a; **4.** d; **5.** You start timing at the beginning of one contraction and continue until the beginning of the next. 6.d. ****Case Study 17.2: 1.** c; **2.** As the baby's head moves through the birth canal, the cord is compressed between the unborn child and the birth canal. Because blood flow to the baby stops, the baby can die from lack of oxygen; 3.b; **4.** F. **Self-Assessment: 1.** b; **2.** d; **3.** c; **4.** c; **5.** c; **6.** a; **7.** d; **8.** b; **9.** a; **10.** b.

Unit 18

Matching: 1. e; **2.** d; **3.** a; **4.** g; **5.** b; **6.** c; **7.** f. **True/False: 1.** F; **2.** T; **3.** F; **4.** T; **5.** F; **6.** T; **7.** T; **8.** F; **9.** T; **10.** F; **11.** F; **12.** T; **13.** T; **14.** T; **15.** F. **Short Answer: 1.** Observe the child before touching him or her. Communicate clearly with the parent or guardian and the child. Remain calm. Do not separate the child from loved ones unless necessary. Gain trust through your actions. **2.** Children are not small adults. A child has unique needs and requires special care. A child does not readily accept strangers. **3.** Fear of the unknown;

fear of being ill or hurt; fear of being touched by strangers; fear of being separated from his or her parents or caregivers. **4.** When opening the airway of an infant or a small child, tilt the head back only enough to have the victim's nose pointing straight up. Place a folded towel under the shoulders to help maintain good airway position. An oral airway can be used to help maintain an open airway if the head-tilt/chin-lift or jaw-thrust maneuver is not effective. **5.** Low blood sugar, poisonings, seizures, infection, trauma, decreased levels of oxygen, and the onset of shock. **6.** An injury that does not fit the description of what caused it; patterns of injury that include cigarette burns, whip marks, and hand prints; obvious or suspected fractures in a child less than 2 years of age; any unexplained fractures; injuries in various stages of healing, especially bruises and burns; unexplained lacerations or abrasions, especially to the mouth, lips, and eyes; injuries to the genitalia; pain when the child sits down; more injuries than are common for a child of the same age; repeated calls to the same address. **7.** Lack of adult supervision; a child who appears to be malnourished; an unsafe living environment; untreated chronic illness, for example, an asthmatic child with no medications. **Case Study 18.1**: **1.** a; **2.** c; **3.** Do a toe-to-head assessment instead of a head-to-toe assessment. Do the toe-to-head assessment before checking vital signs. Keep the child in the car seat while you perform your assessments. **4.** F. **Self- Assessment:** **1.** d; **2.** c; **3.** d; **4.** d; **5.** d; **6.** c; **7.** c; **8.** a; **9.** d; **10.** b.

Unit 19
Matching: **1.** c; **2.** f; **3.** j; **4.** d; **5.** e; **6.** g; **7.** i; **8.** b; **9.** a; **10.** k; **11.** h. **True/False**: **1.** F; **2.** T; **3.** F; **4.** F; **5.** T; **6.** T; **7.** T; **8.** T; **9.** F; **10.** T; **11.** T; **12.** T; **13.** F. **Short Answer**; **1.** A traditional first responder is generally one who functions in the 9-1-1 system. They are usually affiliated with a service. Non-traditional first responders have had the same training as traditional first responders but work in less traditional settings, for example, as athletic trainers or trip leaders. **2.** Airways; suction equipment; artificial ventilation devices, such as resuscitation mask or bag-valve-mask; basic wound supplies, such as dressings and bandages; personal safety equipment, such as gloves and protective eyewear; street maps; scissors; blood pressure cuff and stethoscope; flashlight; note pad and pen; waterless hand washing solution; any other equipment required by local or state standards. **3.** Helicopter and fixed-wing aircraft. **4.** Chocking—blocks or wedges against the wheels; tying the frame to an anchor point with strong rope or chain; letting the air out of all the tires; putting the vehicle in "park," turning off the ignition, and setting the parking brake. **5.** Placards; spilled liquids or solids; unusual odors; clouds of vapors; leaking containers. **Case Study 19.1**: **1.** b; **2.** b; **3.** F; **4.** Burns; Unconsciousness or dazed/confused behavior; respiratory distress or arrest; weak, irregular or absent pulse. **Self-Assessment**: **1.** c; **2.** b; **3.** a; **4.** a; **5.** b; **6.** d; **7.** a; **8.** d; **9.** c; **10.** d; **11.** a.

Notes

Notes

Notes

Notes

Notes

Notes

Notes

MISSION OF THE AMERICAN RED CROSS

The American Red Cross, a humanitarian organization led by volunteers and guided by its Congressional Charter and the Fundamental Principles of the International Red Cross Movement, will provide relief to victims of disaster and help people prevent, prepare for, and respond to emergencies.

ABOUT THE AMERICAN RED CROSS

To support the mission of the American Red Cross, over 1.3 million paid and volunteer staff serve in some 1,600 chapters and blood centers throughout the United States and its territories and on military installations around the world. Supported by the resources of a national organization, they form the largest volunteer service and educational force in the nation. They help people prevent, prepare for, and cope with emergencies, whether those emergencies involve blood, disasters, tissue transplants, social services, or health and safety.

The American Red Cross provides consistent, reliable education and training in injury and illness prevention and emergency care, providing training to nearly 16 million people each year in first aid, CPR, swimming, water safety, and HIV/AIDS education.

All of these essential services are made possible by the voluntary services, blood and tissue donations, and financial support of the American people.

FUNDAMENTAL PRINCIPLES OF THE INTERNATIONAL RED CROSS AND RED CRESCENT MOVEMENT

HUMANITY

IMPARTIALITY

NEUTRALITY

INDEPENDENCE

VOLUNTARY SERVICE

UNITY

UNIVERSALITY